Revitalize & Thrive:

Navigating Menopause with Grace

ISBN: 9798862527308
Imprint: Independently published

To all the remarkable women,

This book is dedicated to you — the architects of strength, the bearers of wisdom, the champions of resilience. Through the highs and lows, the laughter and tears, you've navigated life's labyrinth with unwavering grace.

May these pages serve as a compass, guiding you through the transformative journey of menopause. Just as you've conquered mountains and crossed rivers, you'll conquer this chapter with courage and determination.

In your laughter, may you find freedom. In your tears, may you find healing. In your wisdom, may you find power. In your resilience, may you find hope.

Embrace change, for it is the sculptor of your spirit. Embrace growth, for it is the canvas of your dreams. Embrace yourself, for you are a beacon of light in a world that needs your brilliance.

With every page you turn, remember that your journey is your own, unique and beautiful. You are the author of your narrative, the captain of your ship. May this book empower you to embrace menopause with open arms and a heart full of courage.

To the remarkable women who inspire, uplift, and shine, this book is for you.

With admiration and gratitude,

April

Disclaimer

The information provided in this book, "Revitalize & Thrive: Navigating Menopause with Grace," is intended for general informational purposes only. The content is based on research, personal experiences, and general knowledge available.

While every effort has been made to ensure the accuracy and relevance of the information presented, menopause is a complex and individualized experience. The content in this book should not be considered a substitute for professional medical, psychological, or any other form of advice, diagnosis, or treatment.

Readers are encouraged to consult with qualified healthcare professionals, such as physicians, gynecologists, psychologists, or other experts, to address their specific needs and concerns related to menopause or any other health issues. Medical and psychological conditions can vary widely among individuals, and professional guidance is essential for personalized recommendations and care.

The author, publisher, and any contributors to this book do not assume any responsibility for the accuracy, completeness, or reliability of the information provided herein, nor do they endorse any specific treatments, therapies, or products mentioned in the text. Readers should exercise their own judgment and discretion when applying any information from this book to their personal situations.

By reading this book, you acknowledge and agree that the author, publisher, and contributors are not liable for any direct or indirect consequences that may result from the use of the information contained in this book. Your health and well-being are of paramount importance, and seeking professional advice is crucial for addressing your unique needs.

Remember that health-related information can change over time, and the most current research and guidelines should always be consulted when making important decisions about your health. Your healthcare provider is your best source of guidance and information tailored to your individual circumstances.

Thank you for choosing "Revitalize & Thrive: Navigating Menopause with Grace" as a resource for your menopausal journey. I hope it provides valuable insights and inspires you to prioritize your health and well-being during this transformative phase of life.

Welcome

Hey there, beautiful! I'm April, and I'm thrilled to welcome you to "Revitalize & Thrive: Navigating Menopause with Grace."

Buckle up, because we're about to embark on a journey filled with insights, wisdom, and camaraderie as we navigate the twists and turns of menopause. Why am I so passionate about this topic? Well, because I've walked in your shoes. I've felt the hot flashes, the mood rollercoasters, and the profound changes that menopause can bring, all while being a single parent and trying to build a struggling business. This book is more than just words; it's a heartfelt endeavor to offer you support, empowerment, and a guiding light as you tread through this transformative phase.

Let's be real–menopause isn't just a one-size-fits-all experience. It's unique to each of us, with its own set of challenges and triumphs. And that's where "Revitalize & Thrive: Navigating Menopause with Grace" comes in. As someone who's crossed the threshold into post-menopausal life, I'm honored to be your companion on this journey. From the highs to the hurdles, I'm here to share insights, strategies, and a virtual cup of tea as we navigate this transformative chapter together.

This book is your go-to resource–your trusted confidante–as you embrace the multifaceted world of menopause. Together, we'll explore the nitty-gritty of this phase: from understanding its stages and symptoms to unraveling the mysteries of hormonal changes. But this isn't just about information; it's about empowerment. You'll discover practical tools, self-care techniques, and strategies to reclaim your balance, confidence, and vitality.

Picture this book as a treasure trove–packed with information that honors your body, mind, and spirit. You'll dive into holistic strategies, such as nourishing foods that fuel your well-being, gentle exercises that bring both joy and strength, and mindfulness practices that cultivate inner peace. We'll even venture into the world of holistic remedies that can complement your journey.

Menopause isn't just a biological event; it's a transformative journey that touches every facet of your being. That's why we'll explore everything from self-care rituals that nurture your soul to the power of seeking community support. It's all interconnected-your physical health, emotional resilience, and the beauty of embracing this chapter fully.

So, here's to you–the remarkable woman who's ready to dive into this transformative phase with an open heart and a thirst for knowledge. Through the pages of this book, you'll find not just information, but a roadmap to navigate menopause with grace and resilience. Embrace your journey, dear reader. Together, we're stepping into a world of empowerment, self-discovery, and a celebration of the incredible journey you're embarking upon.

Welcome aboard!

TABLE OF CONTENTS

Introduction:

Hello, my fellow journeyer through the tapestry of life. Today, let's delve into a topic that resonates with every woman: the enigmatic voyage of menopause. It's a phase of life that often comes with a mixture of feelings, and I'm here to be your compass, helping you navigate it with understanding and grace.

Understanding the Menopause Transition

Isn't life an incredible journey? We traverse various chapters, each with its own share of challenges and blessings. Among these transformative phases stands menopause, a unique experience that beckons us to embrace the wisdom it brings. So, let's embark on this exploration, shall we?

Menopause is a natural transition that signals the end of our reproductive years. It typically makes its appearance between our late 40s and early 50s. But remember, there's no strict timeline—it's a personal expedition that unfolds differently for each of us. At its core, menopause is a choreography of hormones. Our ovaries gradually produce less estrogen and progesterone, leading to the closing notes of our menstrual cycles. This hormonal ballet can usher in a range of physical and emotional changes that we'll uncover together.

Here's the fascinating part: no two women dance through menopause in the same way. It's like a canvas awaiting your unique brushstrokes, shaped by your genetics, lifestyle, and health. Some women glide through this phase, barely sensing a shift, while others might encounter more pronounced changes. Remember, this journey is yours, and you're free to travel it at your own rhythm.

Yet, let's not forget the emotional side of this journey. While we often focus on the physical aspects, let's honor the feelings that accompany menopause. It's a whirlwind of emotions, from empowerment to vulnerability. Imagine it as a rollercoaster, each emotion valid and deserving of acknowledgment. By embracing these transitions and seeking support when needed, we grant ourselves permission to bloom fully during this transformation.

As we journey through the upcoming pages, we'll dive into the realm of menopause. From decoding the intricacies of hormonal shifts to uncovering practical strategies to navigate the changes, my aim is to empower you to embrace this phase with grace. Remember, you're never alone on this voyage. Armed with knowledge and a positive outlook, you can sail through this phase with strength and resilience.

Embracing Menopause as a New Life Chapter

Envision life as a captivating novel with countless chapters, each weaving its own story. Menopause beckons us to turn the page, unveiling fresh adventures and uncharted territories. As we step into this chapter, let's approach it as an opportunity for growth, renewal, and self-love.

Embracing menopause as a new life chapter invites us to shed the expectations of society and embrace our authentic selves. It's akin to stepping into your own power, knowing that your worth transcends roles or age. This is your time to shine, to rediscover what sets your soul ablaze, and to craft a life that resonates with your true essence.

Sure, menopause starts change, yet it's also an invitation to connect deeply with your inner self. Embrace your quirks, passions, and the unique tapestry that is you. See this phase as a blank canvas, awaiting your strokes of color — a chance to revisit dreams you might have set aside. By embracing your authentic self, you're sowing seeds for a life brimming with fulfillment.

And let's remember, just as the seasons shift, so do we. Menopause is a reminder that our bodies are resilient and adaptable. It's a time to be thankful for the journey you've traversed, celebrating every step, challenge, and triumph. Embracing the ebb and flow of life allows you to draw strength and courage from within.

As you explore the pages that lie ahead, remember that this is your time to shine. Embrace change, cultivate self-love, and step into this new chapter with excitement. Together, let's celebrate the beauty of menopause as a transformation that enhances our radiance and empowers us even further.

The Importance of Holistic Menopause Management

Imagine a mosaic, each piece contributing to a harmonious whole. This analogy beautifully mirrors how we should approach menopause — holistically. It's about nurturing every facet of our well-being, recognizing that every aspect matters.

Holistic menopause management delves deeper than the surface. It acknowledges that menopause isn't just a physical occurrence; it's a symphony encompassing emotions, thoughts, and spirit. By embracing this holistic perspective, we unlock a treasure trove of tools that nurture every part of us. From the foods we choose to the care we give our minds, it's all interconnected.

The magic of holistic management lies in the art of self-care. It's akin to a loving ritual for your body and soul. By tuning into your body's signals, you're sending a message of compassion and care. It's about choosing foods that nourish you, engaging in activities that bring joy, and finding pockets of tranquility in a bustling world.

Here's the beauty: holistic management doesn't solely focus on physical well-being. It's also about nurturing your inner strength. It's about embracing change and tapping into your innate resilience. By tending to your body, mind, and spirit, you're setting the stage for an empowered journey through menopause and beyond.

In the chapters that lie ahead, we'll uncover the remarkable benefits of holistic menopause management. It's not just about managing symptoms; it's about embarking on a journey of self-discovery, growth, and empowerment that resonates across every facet of your life. So, let's venture forth on this holistic path together, creating a future that radiates with well-being and vitality.

Navigating Menopause with Support and Empowerment

As we navigate the intricate waters of menopause, one thing becomes crystal clear: we're not alone. We are not alone on this journey of menopause, as it is woven into the tapestry of womanhood. It's a time to lean into the support of our community, to share stories, and to uplift one another.

Imagine sitting with your closest friends, cups of soothing tea in hand, as you swap tales of your menopause experiences. The camaraderie that comes from these conversations is priceless. It reminds us we are not the first to sail through these seas, nor will we be the last. We're part of a long line of remarkable women who have traversed this transition before us.

When we open up about our journey, it's incredible how our experiences resonate with others. Sharing the challenges and triumphs creates bonds that transcend age and background. We realize that our unique stories, our insights, and our wisdom have the power to inspire and comfort others. And in return, their stories become a source of strength for us.

In this era of digital connectivity, the online space can also be a sanctuary of understanding. Social media groups and forums are bustling with women who share their menopause experiences openly. These virtual circles can be a haven to ask questions, seek advice, and find kindred spirits who truly understand what you're going through.

Empowerment stems from knowing that you have choices. It's about taking an active role in shaping your menopause journey. Consult with healthcare professionals who specialize in women's health and menopause. They can provide personalized guidance, offer solutions tailored to your needs, and help you make informed decisions about your well-being.

When it comes to managing symptoms, consider a holistic approach that nurtures your body, mind, and spirit. Engage in activities that bring you joy and peace. Explore the world of mindfulness, whether through meditation, deep breathing, or yoga. These practices can be powerful tools to ease the waves of change that menopause brings.

Fostering Self-Love and Acceptance

As we stand at the crossroads of change, it's paramount to cultivate self-love and acceptance. Our bodies have carried us through a lifetime of experiences, and this phase is no different. Treat your body as a cherished friend, one that deserves your utmost care and respect.

Self-love starts with embracing your body, regardless of its changes. Those little quirks and lines are the marks of a life well-lived. Celebrate the wisdom that comes with age, for it's a treasure that only time can bestow. Self-care becomes an act of self-love, a way to honor the vessel that has carried you through life's adventures.

Nourish yourself with wholesome foods that fuel both your body and your spirit. Hydrate, savor the flavors, and relish in the pleasure of eating. Prioritize a balanced diet rich in nutrients that supports bone health, heart health, and overall well-being. Remember, this is a chapter where you invest in yourself.
Movement is another expression of self-love. Engage in physical activities that bring you joy, whether it's dancing, swimming, hiking, or trying a new fitness class. Movement isn't just about staying in shape; it's about feeling alive, vibrant, and connected to your body.

Embracing a Vibrant Future

Picture this: a sunrise casting a warm glow over a new day. This is the energy that embracing menopause can bring to your life—a fresh start filled with possibilities. As you enter this new chapter, consider the dreams that have been whispering to you.

Maybe there's a passion project you've always wanted to pursue—a book to write, an art form to master, or a cause that ignites your soul. With the responsibilities of motherhood and career evolution, you now have the space to focus on these aspirations.

Menopause invites us to redefine ourselves in ways that reflect our true essence. Explore your interests, uncover your talents, and set new goals. You should thrive during this time, chase the dreams that may have been put on hold, and create a legacy that speaks to your unique journey.

When you approach menopause with curiosity and a zest for life, you're opening the door to a future that's not defined by age but by your unyielding spirit. Embrace the adventure, my friend. Your journey is just beginning, and it's filled with chapters of growth, exploration, and a radiance that only deepens with time.

Chapter 1: Menopause Demystified

Hey there friend! Grab a cup of herbal tea and cozy up–we're about to dive into the incredible journey of menopause, and believe me, it's a journey worth embracing with open arms. If you've been feeling like you're on a rollercoaster of emotions and changes, you're not alone. Menopause is like a rite of passage, a journey every woman embarks on. It's not just about hormonal shifts; it's about embracing a new phase of life with grace and empowerment.

I know, I know–those hormones can make you feel like you're on an emotional rollercoaster that just won't stop. One moment you're laughing at a cat video, and the next, you're tearing up over a commercial about laundry detergent. At the extreme, it's like being trapped in a comedy-drama where your emotions have a life of their own.

But let me tell you, dear friend, you're not losing your mind. You're undergoing a profound transformation, one that's been part of the tapestry of womanhood since time immemorial. Menopause is simply a shift, a transition from one stage of life to another, like a caterpillar becoming a butterfly. And just like that caterpillar, you're going through some major changes before you spread your wings and soar.

So lovely soul, let's delve into the world of menopause together, shall we? Picture us sitting in a cozy nook, sharing stories and insights about this transformative phase that's a natural part of every woman's life. Menopause, my dear, is like a bridge connecting our vibrant fertility years to the wisdom-filled chapters that follow. So, let's embark on this journey with curiosity and camaraderie.

Menopause is a remarkable stage in a woman's life, a bit like Mother Nature's gentle way of telling us, "Hey, you've nurtured life within, and now it's time for you to focus on nurturing yourself." It typically takes place between the ages of 45 and 55, although the timing dances uniquely for each of us. At its core, menopause is all about changes in those powerful hormones—estrogen and progesterone—that have been our trusty companions throughout our fertile years.

Imagine your ovaries as star performers in this grand hormonal symphony. As we age, they gradually become less responsive to the signals from our brain, leading to a decrease in the production of eggs. This gracefully leads to the curtain call for our menstrual cycles. Menopause officially takes center stage when you've gone without a period for a year straight, signaling that your ovaries are now on a more tranquil hormonal journey.

But let's not forget about perimenopause, the spirited prelude to menopause. It's like the tango of hormones—sometimes graceful, sometimes unpredictable. During this phase, hormonal shifts can be quite the spectacle, resulting in irregular cycles and a variety of physical and emotional symptoms. You might experience those infamous hot flashes that sweep over you like a warm breeze, followed by night sweats that can turn your cozy bed into a sauna.

Oh, and mood swings! Can we talk about those? Your emotions might feel like a rollercoaster, and trust me, you're not alone. Fluctuating hormones can play tricks on our brain chemistry, causing feelings of irritability, anxiety, and even a hint of the blues. And let's not even mention those sleep disturbances. Tossing and turning like a leaf caught in a summer breeze can become all too familiar.

Now, let's chat about those intimate changes. The hormonal shift might lead to vaginal dryness and changes in libido. It's like your body's way of encouraging new conversations about pleasure and intimacy. Weight gain and metabolism changes can also make a cameo appearance, but remember, your body is just adjusting to this new phase—be patient and kind to yourself.

Keep in mind, my friend, that while these symptoms might sound like a whirlwind, every woman's journey is uniquely her own. It's like a beautiful tapestry woven from the threads of genetics, lifestyle, and overall health. Embracing this transformation allows us to rewrite the narrative—rather than something to fear, menopause can be a time of renewal and rediscovery.

So, what exactly is happening inside your body? Well, let's take a little peek behind the curtain of hormones. Hormones are like the conductors of your body's orchestra. They regulate everything from your sleep patterns to your mood swings. And during menopause, this orchestra is going through a bit of a remix.

Estrogen, the hormone that's been a loyal companion throughout your reproductive years, takes a step back. It's like the diva of the show deciding to go on vacation. And while estrogen's sipping Piña coladas on a beach somewhere, your body is figuring out how to manage without its star player.

This shift can lead to a whole symphony of symptoms–from the infamous hot flashes that make you feel like you're auditioning for a part in a sauna commercial, to night sweats that turn your cozy bed into a slip 'n slide. And let's not forget those mood swings that can make you feel like you're on a rollercoaster of emotions, without a seatbelt.

Let's explore the three major acts of this beautiful play: perimenopause, menopause, and post-menopause.

1. Perimenopause: Now, let's talk about perimenopause-the prelude to the grand symphony of menopause. Think of it as a sneak preview of the main event. During perimenopause, your body is like a wizard's laboratory, experimenting with hormones and giving you a taste of what's to come. This stage can start in your late 30s or early 40s, making you feel like you've stumbled into a hormonal wonderland.

Imagine waking up one day feeling like a superhero, ready to conquer the world. The next day, you're convinced you're auditioning for the role of Grumpy Cat's understudy. Perimenopause can be a bit like that-an unpredictable journey where your hormones decide to play their own version of hide and seek.

Your menstrual cycle, which once resembled a reliable clock, now resembles a Jackson Pollock painting-a beautiful chaos of irregularity. Some months, your period might be fashionably late, while others it arrives unannounced like a surprise guest. It's like your uterus is throwing a party, and it can't decide on the guest list.

And then there are the symptoms that show up like uninvited guests. Hot flashes, those sudden bursts of warmth that feel like your body's auditioning for the sun, become a regular occurrence. You might find yourself fanning yourself in the dead of winter or waking up in the middle of the night feeling like you've been placed in an oven.

Oh, and let's not forget the mood swings. It's like your emotions are on a seesaw, and someone keeps adding sandbags to one side.

But here's the silver lining–perimenopause isn't just a series of inconvenient symptoms. It's also an opportunity for growth and self-discovery. Just like a caterpillar in its cocoon, you're undergoing a transformation. You're shedding old patterns, redefining your priorities, and learning to listen to the whispers of your body.

During perimenopause, self-care becomes your trusty companion. Remember, you're not just a caretaker for others; you're the guardian of your own well-being. It's about setting boundaries, prioritizing rest, and embracing practices that nourish your body and soul.

2. Menopause: Now, let's talk about menopause–the main event, the grand finale, the point in the journey where your body and hormones march to a different beat. If perimenopause was the preview, menopause is the opening act of this transformative performance.

Imagine a world where your periods, those monthly visitors that brought a mixed bag of cramps and cravings, are now bidding you adieu. Yes, you heard that right–no more stocking up on feminine hygiene products or timing your life around the menstrual calendar. It's like waving goodbye to an old friend, and while there might be a hint of nostalgia, there's also a sense of relief.

But let's talk about the stars of the menopause show–the infamous hot flashes. You know the drill: one moment, you're feeling perfectly comfortable, and the next, your body is a furnace. It's like an internal thermostat gone rogue, turning up the heat without your permission. Your cheeks flush, your skin tingles, and suddenly, you're contemplating setting up camp in the freezer aisle of your local grocery store.

And while we're on the topic of temperature regulation, let's not forget the night sweats. Picture waking up drenched, your pyjamas clinging to your skin like a second layer. It's as if your body decided to host a tropical rainforest adventure in the middle of your sleep. You're left tossing, turning, and cursing the overzealous radiator that is your hormonal system.

But here's the kicker–menopause isn't just about physical changes. It's a symphony of shifts that extends to the emotional realm as well. Mood swings, those unpredictable surges of emotions, become your uninvited companions. One moment, you're as content as a cat lounging in the sun, and the next, you're grappling with a surge of frustration that came out of nowhere.

However, amidst all these changes, there's a silver lining. Menopause isn't a signal that life's adventures are over. No, quite the opposite! It's an invitation to embrace the wisdom you've gained over the years and channel it into new endeavors. It's about rediscovering your passions, embracing your newfound freedom, and connecting with the vibrant woman you've become.

3. Post-Menopause: Now, let's talk about post-menopause – the encore, the aftermath, when the hormonal storm starts to settle, revealing the beautifully transformed landscape of your life. If perimenopause was the prelude and menopause was the crescendo, post-menopause is the serene aftermath where you can bask in the glow of your journey.

Picture this: you wake up one day, and the hot flashes have become distant memories, like old photographs tucked away in a dusty album. Your body's internal thermostat has finally learned to keep its cool. The once-frequent night sweats are now as rare as a shooting star, leaving you to enjoy uninterrupted slumber and wake up feeling refreshed.

But the real magic of post-menopause lies in the emotional realm. Remember those mood swings that used to play havoc with your emotions? They're like long-lost acquaintances you're meeting at a reunion, and you can't help but chuckle at the memories they bring back. You've gained a sense of emotional balance that's akin to sipping herbal tea on a tranquil morning.

Post-menopause is like stepping into the sunlight after a stormy night. Your perspective shifts, and suddenly, you're seeing life through a new lens. It's a phase where you can redefine your priorities, explore uncharted territories, and embark on adventures that were once just distant dreams.

One of the most empowering aspects of post-menopause is the freedom that comes with it. You're no longer bound by the monthly rhythms of your menstrual cycle, giving you the opportunity to reclaim your time and energy. It's like shedding layers of obligations and expectations, allowing your authentic self to shine through.

And let's not forget the sense of wisdom that accompanies this phase. You've weathered the storms of hormonal shifts and emerged on the other side stronger and wiser. Your experiences are etched in the lines on your face, the grace in your movements, and the depth of your laughter. You've earned every inch of your journey, and you wear it with pride.

The period after menopause isn't solely about the person. It's a time to nurture and deepen relationships, to cultivate a sense of sisterhood with other women who've journeyed through the same valleys and peaks. It's a chapter where you can share your stories, listen to others, and create a tapestry of collective wisdom.

So, my fellow traveler, as we explore the landscapes of post-menopause, remember that this phase is like a reward for the journey you've taken. You're not just entering a new chapter; you're stepping into a world of possibility and potential. In the chapters that follow, we'll delve deeper into the joys and opportunities that post-menopause brings.

This journey is about nourishing yourself in every sense of the word. It's about finding harmony through nutrition, movement, mindfulness, and even a dash of laughter. Because let's face it–laughing at the absurdity of life's twists and turns can be incredibly cathartic.

In the chapters that follow, we'll dive deeper into the realms of nutrition, exercise, managing your mood, getting quality sleep, and embracing complementary therapies. We'll tackle body image with love and care, explore the dynamics of relationships and intimacy, and discover the exciting opportunities that lie beyond menopause.

Let's raise our cups of herbal tea to this adventure. Let's embrace the changes, celebrate the small victories, and journey forward with a heart full of curiosity and courage. Because menopause isn't an end–it's a breathtaking beginning.

Remember, dear friend, you're not alone on this journey. Seeking support from friends, family, and healthcare professionals can make all the difference. As you navigate the waves of change, embrace your newfound wisdom and celebrate the woman you've become. Menopause is a reminder that you're a force of nature, capable of embracing every chapter of life with grace and resilience. Here's to the journey ahead, and to you—radiant, powerful, and ready to embrace it all. Cheers to menopause!

Chapter 2: Hormonal Changes and Your Body

Hormones and Their Role in Menopause

Hey girlfriend! Let's dive into the secret world of hormones–those tiny powerhouses that have been orchestrating our lady business since day one. You know, those mood swings, cramps, and cravings? Yep, hormones are the conductors behind the scenes. And when it comes to menopause, these hormonal maestros take center stage, conducting a symphony of change that can leave us feeling like we're on an emotional rollercoaster.

Now, picture this: hormones are like our body's personal DJs. They've got the playlist for every stage of life, and menopause is like their remix–a mixtape of physical and emotional changes that can leave us saying, "Wait, who invited you to the party?"

First up, we have estrogen–the VIP hormone that's been holding down the fort since our teenage years. It's the one responsible for our monthly dance with Aunt Flo, setting the stage for ovulation and keeping everything in sync. But guess what? When menopause steps in, estrogen plays the quiet game. It's like our ovary's star player is taking a vacation, and we're left with fewer ovulations and some interesting side effects.

Then there's progesterone–our wing woman in the reproductive show. It's like estrogen's partner in crime, getting our uterine lining all ready for a potential bun in the oven. But as menopause enters, progesterone's attendance dwindles. And that, my friend, is the closing act for our fertile years.

But wait, there's more! We've got FSH and LH–the hormones that could win the award for "Most Likely to Make You Feel Like You're Losing Your Mind!" Produced in our brain's pituitary gland, these two work together to keep our menstrual cycle in check. But when menopause knocks on the door, FSH and LH go into overdrive, trying to jumpstart our ovaries like they're revving an old engine.

And here's a twist–testosterone, the hormone we usually associate with guys, is also hanging out in our system, albeit in smaller amounts. It's like that cool cousin who shows up unexpectedly to the family gathering. Testosterone keeps our libido in check and adds a dash of wellness to the mix. But as menopause throws its hat in the ring, testosterone's party might get a little quieter.

Now, let's talk about symptoms–the real MVPs of menopause. Hot flashes that make you feel like a human torch? Check. Night sweats that turn your bed into a slip 'n slide? Oh, absolutely. Mood swings that leave you crying over a cute puppy video? Yep, those too. It's like our hormones are having a field day, and we're along for the ride.

But here's the thing: menopause isn't a one-size-fits-all kind of deal. The journey is as unique as we are. So, while we might share the spotlight with these hormonal shifts, the way we dance to their tune is our own special rhythm.

Understanding this hormonal tango is like having a secret map for this journey. It helps us navigate the highs, the lows, and everything in between. And guess what? Menopause isn't a finale; it's an encore. It's an invitation to put ourselves first, explore new ways to handle these changes, and step into this next chapter of life with a big ol' dose of grace and strength.

So, let's raise our cups of herbal tea to this adventure, my friend. Let's embrace the changes, celebrate the victories, and dance through menopause like the rock stars we are.

Riding the Hormonal Waves - Navigating Physical and Emotional Changes

Hey, girl, let's get real about those hormonal rollercoasters our bodies love to take us on. Hormones? Oh yeah, they're like our body's secret sauce, spicing up our physical and emotional journey through life. And let me tell you, nowhere is their impact more in-your-face than during the wild ride called menopause.

Physically, it's like hormones are our backstage crew, working their magic (or mischief). You know those hot flashes that hit you out of nowhere, making you feel like you're sunbathing in Antarctica? Yeah, those. They mess with your sleep, leaving you as energized as a half-drained battery. Blame it on the declining estrogen levels–it's like our internal thermostat got a memo to go haywire.

And let's not forget the night sweats. Your bed becomes a swimming pool, and you're the reluctant lifeguard. But guess what? These sleep disturbances are like tag-along friends with mood swings. Yep, mood swings. They're the unexpected guests at the party, making you go from laughter to tears faster than you can say "chocolate."

Speaking of hormones messing with us, the drop in estrogen during menopause isn't just playing around. It's like the foundation of a house getting a little shaky. Our bones weaken, putting us at risk for osteoporosis and fractures. And if that's not enough, hormones mess with our metabolism and where we store those pesky pounds. Weight management turns into a game of hide and seek.

But hold on, because the emotional dance isn't over. Hormones can turn our feelings into a rollercoaster playlist. Mood swings become our new roommates, and suddenly, irritability, sadness, and feeling like a raw nerve are all part of our emotional playlist. Anxiety can waltz in uninvited too, adding another layer to the mix.

But hey, sister, it's crucial to remember that while hormones might be the headliners, they're not the entire show. Our genes, life experiences, and the support we have around us play their parts too. It's like a big ensemble cast shaping our emotional scenes.

And here's the thing–this hormonal theater isn't just happening to us. We're not simply bystanders, we hold the power to act. We can approach these changes with compassion and a dash of proactive magic. Exercise becomes our superhero cape, a balanced diet our ally, stress-reduction techniques our secret weapons, and seeking emotional support our knight in shining armor. And let's not forget the holistic approach–that's like our personal treasure map to navigate this adventure.

So, my amazing friend, let's embrace these hormonal waves. Let's give ourselves permission to ride the ups and downs with grace and understanding. We're the leading ladies of this show, and we've got the power to make menopause a chapter full of strength, self-love, and unstoppable spirit.

Finding Your Hormonal Harmony - Embracing Natural Strategies

Let's chat about something that's the talk of the town–hormones and how to keep them in line during the menopause marathon. You know, that wild ride where hormones seem to have a mind of their own? Well, I've got some insider tips that can help you find your own groove and sail through this transformative journey.

Now, picture this: we're on a quest for hormonal balance, and it's like searching for that missing earring in a messy room. Menopause throws our hormones into a whirlwind, and suddenly, our bodies are speaking a new language. While there are medical options on the table, a lot of us are eyeing the natural path to help our bodies find their rhythm again.

So, what's the deal with these natural strategies? They're like our secret weapons–they empower us to take the reins of our health and make menopause our own story. And trust me, it's like stepping into a power suit and saying, "Hey hormones, I've got this!"

Nutrition and Diet: Let's talk diet–it's not about crazy restrictions, but about giving our body the VIP treatment. Foods rich in omega-3 fatty acids, like salmon and chia seeds, are like a backstage pass to hormonal harmony. And guess what? Whole grains, leafy greens, and colorful veggies? They're like our hormone's BFFs, cheering them on to do their best dance.

A balanced and nutrient-rich diet forms the foundation for hormonal balance. Incorporating whole foods, such as fruits, vegetables, whole grains, lean proteins, and healthy fats, provides essential nutrients that support hormone production and regulation. Phytoestrogen-rich foods like flaxseeds, soy, and legumes may help mimic estrogen's effects in the body. Reducing processed foods, sugars, and excessive caffeine can also contribute to stable hormone levels.

Regular Exercise: Exercise? Oh, that's our personal dance party. Cardio and strength training? They're like our personal cheerleaders, releasing those feel-good endorphins and telling our hormones, "You've got this, girl!"

Engaging in regular physical activity has a positive impact on hormone balance. Exercise can help manage weight, reduce stress, and improve mood. Aerobic exercises like walking, jogging, and dancing, as well as strength training and yoga, can all contribute to a healthier hormonal profile. Aim for at least 150 minutes of moderate-intensity exercise per week.

Stress Management: And then there's the relaxation game. Stress-reduction techniques, like yoga and deep breathing, are like our calming mentors, teaching us to slow down and find our Zen.

Chronic stress can disrupt hormone balance, exacerbating menopause symptoms. Practicing stress-reduction techniques such as deep breathing, meditation, mindfulness, and progressive muscle relaxation can help regulate cortisol levels and promote emotional well-being. Engaging in activities that bring joy and relaxation, such as hobbies and spending time in nature, can also contribute to stress reduction.

Adequate Sleep: Quality sleep? It's like the magic spell for hormonal harmony–think of it as a rejuvenation potion for our body and mind.

Prioritizing sleep is essential for hormone balance. Aim for 7-9 hours of quality sleep per night. Create a sleep-conducive environment by keeping the bedroom cool, dark, and quiet. Establishing a consistent sleep schedule and practicing relaxation techniques before bedtime can improve sleep quality and support hormonal health.

Emotional Wellness: But hold on, because we're not just talking about physical stuff here. Emotional wellness? That's like our soul's spa day. Surrounding ourselves with positivity, practicing gratitude, and staying connected with loved ones? They're like our emotional superheroes, helping us keep our cool through the hormonal rollercoaster.

Herbal Supplements: Certain herbal supplements have been used traditionally to support hormone balance. Black cohosh, dong quai, evening primrose oil, and chaste berry are among the botanical options that some women find beneficial. Consult a healthcare provider before incorporating herbal supplements into your regimen, especially if you have pre-existing medical conditions or are taking medications.

Mindful Lifestyle Choices: Reducing exposure to environmental toxins, such as chemicals found in household products and pesticides, can contribute to hormone balance. Opt for natural and organic alternatives when possible. Avoiding excessive alcohol consumption and quitting smoking can support overall health and hormonal equilibrium.

And the best part? These natural strategies aren't just quick fixes; they're like tools we can carry with us on this journey and beyond. They're our secret potion for empowerment, helping us make menopause a chapter of strength, self-love, and unbreakable spirit.

It's important to note that natural strategies for balancing hormones may take time to yield noticeable results. Every woman's body is unique, and finding the right combination of approaches that work for you may require experimentation and patience. Consulting with a healthcare provider or a qualified holistic practitioner can provide personalized guidance and support as you embark on your journey to hormonal balance during menopause.

Chapter 3: Nutrition and Diet for Menopause

Nourishing Your Body - The Power of Nutrient-Rich Foods

Hey, my fellow goddess, on this menopause journey! Let's dive deep into something that's like your secret weapon against all the twists and turns–the magic of nutrient-rich foods. You know, those goodies that not only satisfy our taste buds but also give our body that extra love it deserves during this transformative phase. So, grab your cup of herbal tea, and let's chat about why these foods are like our VIP pass to rock this menopause show.

Okay, picture this: our bodies are like these intricate machines going through a renovation. Menopause throws in its own kind of magic, and suddenly, we're not speaking the same nutritional language as before. But don't fret, because nutrient-rich foods are like our translator, helping us navigate these changes like the queens we are.

Let's start with hormone balance–oh yeah, the symphony of our bodies. Nutrient-rich foods are like the notes that keep everything in tune. Ever heard of phytoestrogens? They're like the plant-based superheroes found in soy, flaxseeds, and whole grains. These little wonders mimic estrogen, keeping those hormones in check. And guess what? Say goodbye to some of the menopause drama like hot flashes and mood swings.

Now, bone health–it's like building our fortress. Menopause might throw some curveballs, but nutrient-rich foods are our armor. Calcium, vitamin D, vitamin K, and magnesium? They're like the knights guarding our precious bones. Think dairy or plant-based alternatives, leafy greens, nuts, seeds, and even fatty fish. They're our allies against the risk of osteoporosis and fractures.

And hello, heart health–because we deserve a happy heart. Nutrient-rich foods are like our heart's besties, keeping it in tip-top shape. Fruits, veggies, whole grains, lean proteins, and those yummy healthy fats? They're like the heart's secret stash. They manage our cholesterol levels, blood pressure, and that overall heart glow. And don't forget about omega-3 fatty acids–they're like the peacekeepers, calming inflammation and making our heart dance with joy.

Now, let's talk weight management–because our bodies are our canvas. Menopause might try to add some extra brushstrokes, but nutrient-rich foods are like the skilled artist. Veggies, fruits, and whole grains? They're like the palette that satisfies our hunger while keeping the calories in check. And protein? It's like the sculptor, preserving our lean muscles and giving our metabolism a high-five.

And guess what, lovely? Our emotions matter too. Nutrient-rich foods are like our emotional cheerleaders. B vitamins, omega-3s, and those antioxidants? They're like the boosters for our mood and emotional well-being. That rainbow of fruits, vibrant veggies, whole grains, and the glorious fatty fish? They're like our positivity potion, giving us that radiant outlook and emotional resilience.

But remember, gorgeous, our bodies are unique, and our nutritional needs are like fingerprints. Menopause might change the rules, but we're still the queens of our kingdom. So, let's cherish these nutrient-rich foods like the gifts they are. They're our lifeline, helping us rock this menopause stage with vitality, strength, and all the sparkle we've got inside.

Eating Your Way through Menopause - What to Dig into and What to Pass on

Hey there, beautiful soul! Let's pull up a chair and have a heart-to-heart about something that's like the magic wand for your menopause journey — the food we put on our plate. Yep, those delicious bites can be our allies, helping us breeze through this phase with a smile. So, grab your favorite snack, and let's chat about what to embrace and what to give a polite nod to during this incredible ride.

Okay, picture this: our bodies are like canvases, and the foods we choose are like the paintbrush strokes. Menopause is this whirlwind artist, and suddenly, our body's needs are singing a new tune. But don't worry, because we've got the ultimate menu plan to make sure our bodies are getting all the love they need.

Let's talk about the heroes of the plate–the foods to include. Fiber-rich buddies like whole grains, fruits, and veggies? They're like our digestive fairy godmothers. They keep things moving and help us feel like a million bucks. Oh, and let's not forget the superstar protein–it's like our body's repair crew, keeping our muscles strong and metabolism on point.

Now, let's give a round of applause for those omega-3 fatty acids. Found in fatty fish, walnuts, and flaxseeds, they're like

our anti-inflammatory warriors. They dance with our heart
and make sure it's singing the happiest tunes.
And speaking of the heart, let's give a warm welcome to our
plant-based friends–the legumes and nuts. They're like our
heart's BFFs, waving away bad cholesterol and keeping our
ticker in check.

Now, the part we all love–antioxidants. They're like our secret
age-defying agents, found in berries, leafy greens, and colorful
veggies. These little wonders combat free radicals and keep
our skin glowing and our cells happy.

But wait, let's talk about the not-so-welcome guests–the foods
to avoid. Refined sugars and processed treats? They're like
those party crashers who bring negativity to the bash. They
mess with our energy levels and mood swings, and girl, we're
here to party with positivity.

Salty foods? They're like the drama queens of our plate. They
mess with our fluid balance and can lead to bloating and
discomfort, like an unwanted guest who overstays their
welcome.

And let's not forget about the caffeine overload. While a cup
of coffee is our morning hug, too much caffeine can be like
that wild friend who keeps us up all night. It messes with our
sleep and can trigger hot flashes — not the adventure we're
after.

So, my amazing friend, let's make this menopause journey a
delicious one. Think of your plate as your canvas, and these
foods as your masterpieces. Embrace the heroes, wave
goodbye to the not-so-greats, and craft a menu that's like a
love letter to your body. Because you, my dear, are worth
every bite.

Foods to Include:

1. Whole Grains: Incorporate whole grains like quinoa, brown rice, oats, and whole wheat to provide sustained energy and stabilize blood sugar levels. Whole grains are rich in fiber, which aids digestion and helps manage weight.

2. Fruits and Vegetables: Colorful fruits and vegetables are rich in antioxidants, vitamins, and minerals that support immune function and reduce inflammation. These nutrient powerhouses contribute to heart health, bone strength, and emotional well-being.

3. Plant-Based Protein: Legumes (beans, lentils, and chickpeas), tofu, tempeh, and nuts provide plant-based protein that supports muscle health, metabolism, and satiety. Including these protein sources can be beneficial for managing weight and promoting overall health.

4. Fatty Fish: Salmon, mackerel, and sardines are high in omega-3 fatty acids, which have anti-inflammatory properties and support heart and brain health. Omega-3s may also help ease mood swings and promote emotional well-being.

5. Healthy Fats: Avocados, nuts, seeds, and olive oil provide healthy fats that support hormone production and absorption of fat-soluble vitamins. These fats contribute to skin health, brain function, and cardiovascular health.

6. Fiber-Rich Foods: Foods high in fiber, such as beans, whole grains, fruits, and vegetables, promote digestive health and regulate bowel movements. Adequate fiber intake can help ease digestive discomfort during menopause.

Foods to Avoid or Limit:

1. Processed and Sugary Foods: Highly processed foods, sugary snacks, and sweetened beverages can lead to blood sugar spikes and crashes, exacerbating mood swings and energy fluctuations. These foods can also contribute to weight gain.

2. Caffeine and Alcohol: Excessive caffeine consumption may worsen sleep disturbances and anxiety. While moderate alcohol consumption can be included, excessive alcohol intake may disrupt sleep and contribute to weight gain.

3. Salty Foods: High sodium intake can contribute to bloating, water retention, and increased blood pressure. Reducing salt intake can help manage these symptoms and promote heart health.

4. Fried and Greasy Foods: Foods high in unhealthy fats may contribute to weight gain and inflammation. Limiting fried and greasy foods can support cardiovascular health and overall well-being.

5. Spicy Foods: Spicy foods may trigger or worsen hot flashes and night sweats in some women. Reducing the consumption of heavily spiced dishes may help manage these symptoms.

But here's the thing, darling–your journey is unique, and your body has its own set of preferences. So, when it comes to crafting your plate, it's all about listening to those cues. Your body knows what it wants, and a little help from a healthcare provider or a registered dietitian can be like a magic wand guiding you through your choices.

So, let's make your menopause experience deliciously yours. Your plate? It's like a canvas for you to paint your vitality and strength. Fill it with love, listen to your body, and watch how those bites become your partners in this incredible adventure.

Let's Dig In - Nourishing Your Body with Deliciousness

Hey there, foodie friend! Grab your fork and let's have a chat about something that's pure joy–our meal plans. Yep, those scrumptious bites that light up our taste buds and keep our bodies dancing through this menopause journey. So, let's take a peek at some meal magic, shall we?

Alright, imagine this: our plates are like our canvases, and the foods we choose are like the vibrant colors that bring them to life. Menopause is like a whirlwind artist, and suddenly, our taste preferences are doing the tango. But don't worry, because we're about to craft meal plans that are like your personal masterpiece.

Let's start with the heroes of the plate–nutrient-rich goodies. Whole grains? They're like the hearty foundation of your meal, giving you that energy boost to conquer the day. Lean proteins? They're like your body's cheering squad, keeping your muscles strong and your tummy satisfied. And healthy fats? Oh, they're like the cozy blanket that keeps you feeling full and content.

Now, let's raise our cups to the hydration game. Herbal tea, water, and those refreshing sips? They're like your body's best friends, keeping you hydrated and your skin glowing.

Remember, we're aiming for that healthy glow from the inside out.

And guess what? We've got not one, but two sample meal plans to spark your taste buds. In the first plan, we're all about variety. We're talking about oatmeal with berries for breakfast, a colorful salad with grilled chicken for lunch, and baked salmon with veggies for dinner. Snacks? Oh yeah, some almonds and yogurt. It's like a symphony of flavors that your taste buds will dance to.

Now, let's dive into the second plan–a plant-powered delight. Think of a smoothie bowl packed with berries for breakfast, a hearty chickpea and veggie stir-fry for lunch, and a lentil and vegetable curry for dinner. Snacks? How celery with almond butter? It's like a garden of flavors that shows off the deliciousness of plant-based options.

Sample Meal Plan 1: Balanced Day

Breakfast:

- Overnight oats topped with mixed berries, chopped nuts, and a drizzle of honey

- Herbal tea or decaffeinated coffee

Lunch:

- Grilled chicken salad with mixed greens, cherry tomatoes, cucumbers, bell peppers, avocado, and a light vinaigrette
- Quinoa or whole grain roll on the side

Snack:

- Greek yogurt with a sprinkle of ground flaxseeds and a small handful of almonds

Dinner:

- Baked salmon with roasted sweet potatoes and steamed broccoli

- Mixed salad with leafy greens, chickpeas, carrots, and a lemon-tahini dressing

---

Sample Meal Plan 2: Plant-Powered Day

Breakfast:

- Smoothie with spinach, frozen berries, banana, almond milk, chia seeds, and a scoop of plant-based protein powder

Lunch:

- Chickpea and vegetable stir-fry with quinoa

- Sliced oranges for dessert

Snack:

- Celery sticks with almond butter

Dinner:

- Lentil and vegetable curry served over brown rice

- Side salad with mixed greens, bell peppers, cucumber, and a light vinaigrette

But hold on, darling! These plans are like your starting line. Add your own magic–swap ingredients, experiment with flavors, and make it a culinary adventure that you truly enjoy. Remember, it's all about making your taste buds sing and your body dance with happiness.

And when in doubt, consult with a registered dietitian. They're like your personal meal whisperers, helping you align your choices with your health goals and those little menopause-related concerns.

Chapter 4: Exercise and Fitness for Hormonal Health

Let's Get Moving - Unleash Your Inner Exercise Diva

Hey there, my fellow fabulous warrior! It's time to lace up those sneakers and have a heart-to-heart about something that's like your secret weapon against the menopause whirlwind–exercise. Yep, those moves you make can be your superpower, helping you rock this transformative phase like the queen you are. So, let's grab that water bottle and dive into the world of fitness magic!

Imagine this: your body is like this incredible vessel, and exercise is the fuel that keeps it sailing smoothly. Menopause is like that gust of change, and suddenly, your body's needs are having a little dance party. But guess what? You're about to throw on your dancing shoes and join in!

Let's talk about the magic of exercise – it's like your daily dose of happy pills. Feeling low? Exercise releases those endorphins, and suddenly, your mood is doing the cha-cha. Plus, those sweat sessions? They're like your personal stress busters, waving goodbye to those worries.

Now, let's give a high-five to your bones. Menopause might throw a few curveballs, but exercise is like their superhero protector. Weight-bearing exercises? They're like your bone's best buddies, keeping them strong and ready to take on the world.

And oh, heart health! Exercise is like your heart's love language. Cardio workouts? They're like your heart's dance party, keeping it in top-notch shape. Blood pressure? It's like a student in your fitness class, learning to behave itself and stay in line.

But guess what? Exercise isn't just about the physical. It's like a magical potion for your brain, too. It improves your focus, sharpens your memory, and leaves you feeling like the smartest kid in the class. And let's not forget about that body confidence–exercise is like your personal cheerleader, reminding you that you're strong and beautiful.

So, how do you unleash this exercise diva within you? It's all about finding something you love. Whether it's dancing, yoga, hiking, or hitting the gym, the choice is yours. It's not about being perfect; it's about moving, sweating, and embracing the journey.

And here's the secret ingredient–consistency. Regular exercise is like a promise you make to yourself. It's a date with your body, a commitment to your well-being, and a celebration of your strength.

Physical Health:

1. Bone Health: Weight-bearing exercises like walking, jogging, dancing, and strength training help promote bone density and reduce the risk of osteoporosis. Strong bones are essential for preventing fractures and maintaining mobility.

Weight-bearing exercises? They're like the knights that protect your precious bones. Walking? It's like your daily stroll through the castle gardens. Jogging? It's like your sprint to defend your fortress. Dancing? Oh, that's like your grand ball, where your bones get to mingle and strengthen. And strength training? It's like your armory, giving you the tools to fight against osteoporosis and keep those bones unbreakable.

Strong bones aren't just about avoiding fractures; they're about maintaining your freedom to move. It's like telling your body, "Hey, we're not slowing down–we're just getting started!"

So, what's the secret to unlocking this bone warrior within you? It's all about finding moves that make you feel alive. Whether it's a brisk walk in the morning, a dance-off in your living room, or lifting weights like a total boss, the choice is yours. It's not about being the fastest or the strongest; it's about being the best version of you.

And let's not forget–consistency is your trusty sidekick. Regular exercise isn't just a routine; it's a pact you make with your body. It's like saying, "I've got your back, bones. We're in this together!"

So, my incredible friend, lace up those shoes and step into your power. Menopause might knock on the door, but you've got the key to a fortress that's unbreakable. Your bones are your allies, and every step, every dance, every move you make is a reminder that you're strong, you're fierce, and you're ready to conquer anything that comes your way.

2. Weight Management: Menopause can bring about changes in metabolism and weight distribution. Regular exercise helps manage weight by burning calories, preserving lean muscle mass, and promoting a healthy body composition.

3. Heart Health: Aerobic activities, such as swimming, cycling, and brisk walking, support cardiovascular health by improving circulation, lowering blood pressure, and reducing the risk of heart disease. Exercise contributes to healthier cholesterol levels and overall heart function.

Shine Bright - Nurturing Your Mental and Emotional Well-being

Hey, soul sister! It's time to dive into something that's like your personal potion of joy — your mental and emotional well-being. Yep, those feelings you carry and the thoughts that twirl in your mind, they deserve some love too. So, grab a cozy blanket, let's cozy up, and chat about how to keep your heart and mind shining through this menopause journey.

Imagine this: your mind is like a garden, and exercise is like the water that helps those beautiful thoughts bloom. Menopause is like that whirlwind friend who's rearranging your thoughts, and suddenly, your emotions are having a little dance-off. But guess what? You're about to jump into that dance, and it's all going to be spectacular.

Let's start with stress—it's like that rain cloud that needs a little sunshine. Exercise? It's like your sunshine, banishing those cortisol clouds and bringing in those feel-good vibes. When you move, those magical endorphins are released, and suddenly, your stress melts away, leaving you feeling lighter than air.

Now, let's talk about mood — it's like the colors of your heart. Regular exercise is like your paintbrush, adding hues of happiness and swiping away those shades of blue. Depression? Anxiety? Well, they're like the weeds in your garden, and exercise? It's like your ultimate gardener, pulling them out and leaving behind a garden of positivity.

And how about that brainpower? It's like your secret library of wisdom. Exercise is like your librarian, keeping the shelves neat and organized. Blood flow to the brain? It's like the nourishment your mind craves, keeping your thoughts sharp and your memory sparkling. Physical activity has been known to boost cognitive function, memory, and clarity, making sure you're the smartest cookie in the jar.

So, how do you light up your mental and emotional wellness? It's all about moving in ways that make your heart happy. Whether it's a calming yoga session, a powerful run, or even a dance party in your living room, the choice is yours. It's not about perfection; it's about progress and those little moments of joy.

Embrace Every Moment - Elevating Your Quality of Life

Hey, kindred spirit! Let's have a heart-to-heart about something that's like the treasure map to a life well-lived — your quality of life. Yep, those moments that fill your heart, the sleep that wraps you in dreams, and the energy that makes you feel alive, they're all part of this incredible journey. So, snuggle into your comfiest spot, and let's dive into the world of embracing life's magic through menopause and beyond.

Imagine this: your life is like a collection of beautiful snapshots, and exercise is like the brush that adds those vibrant strokes. Menopause is like that wise friend who's showing you new perspectives, and suddenly, your quality of life is getting a makeover. But guess what? You're about to grab that brush and create a masterpiece that's uniquely yours.

Let's talk about the dreamland—sleep. It's like that cozy sanctuary where you find rest. Exercise? It's like your lullaby, soothing your mind and inviting sweet dreams to dance in. Menopause might play a little sleep trick, but regular physical activity? It's like your bedtime story, leading you to more restful nights and those oh-so-precious mornings where you wake up feeling refreshed.

Now, how about energy? It's like your personal fuel for life's adventures. Menopause might throw in a few energy dips, but exercise? It's like your superhero cape, sweeping in and banishing those feelings of sluggishness. When you move, it's like your body's wake-up call—suddenly, you're ready to conquer the day with a spirit that's unstoppable.

But wait, there's more! It's about that sense of empowerment—the feeling that you're the captain of your ship. Exercise is like your compass, guiding you towards accomplishments and achievements. Every step you take, every milestone you reach, it's like a nod from the universe, saying, "You've got this!" It's a reminder that you're capable, strong, and you're writing your own story.

So, how do you elevate your quality of life? It's all about choosing moves that light up your heart. Whether it's a sunrise walk, a dance class that brings out your inner diva, or even a gentle yoga session, the choice is yours. It's not about competition; it's about connection — to your body, to your soul, and to the moments that make life truly worth living.

Embracing regular exercise during menopause is an investment in one's physical and emotional well-being. Starting with activities that align with individual preferences and fitness levels and gradually progressing can pave the way for sustainable habits. Consulting with a healthcare provider before beginning an exercise routine is recommended, especially if there are pre-existing medical conditions. By incorporating exercise into the daily routine, women can harness its transformative power and reap the multitude of benefits it offers throughout the menopause journey and beyond.

Customizing Your Exercise Journey - Tailoring Workouts to Tackle Menopause Challenges

So, here's the deal — exercise is like that versatile tool in your toolkit. It's not one-size-fits-all; it's more like that comfy sweater you wear on different occasions. Menopause? Well, it's like that art class where you're painting your own masterpiece. And the right exercises? They're your colors, helping you add those vibrant strokes to your canvas of well-being.

Let's start with the menopause showstopper — hot flashes and night sweats. Imagine this as your cooling fan. Brisk walks, swims that make you feel like a mermaid, or cycling adventures — they're like your superheroes against those fiery flashes. And oh, the relaxation magic of yoga and deep breaths? They're like your secret weapons, taming stress like a boss and keeping the heat at bay.

Now, let's talk about mood swings — those unexpected gusts in the emotional weather forecast. Picture jogging or dancing as your mood lifters. They're like a dance party for your brain, releasing those endorphins and making your mood do a happy jig. And hey, mind-body buddies like tai chi and mindfulness? They're like your emotional anchors, keeping you steady and balanced amid the storm.

Next up? Weight management—like your sculpting session at the gym. Imagine cardio like jogging or cycling as your fat-burning bonfire, while strength training like weightlifting builds those sleek muscles. It's like having your very own metabolism boosters, ensuring your body's engine keeps running smoothly.

And bones? They're like your lifelong companions. Activities like hiking, dancing, or stair climbing? They're like the bone-building architects, creating a firm foundation. Strength training? It's like your blueprint for durability, giving your bones the power to withstand anything.

Sleep issues? Oh, they're like that midnight puzzle. Regular exercise, of any kind, is like your sleep savior. But remember, avoid the superhero moves right before bed; they might keep you up past your bedtime. Instead, embrace gentle yoga or stretching—they're like your lullabies, preparing you for a serene slumber.

Now, here's the twist—your exercise journey should be as unique as your fingerprint. It's about picking what you love, what fits your life, and what feels like a warm hug for your body. Whether it's a dance-off in your living room, a morning jog that makes your heart sing, or a calming yoga session, it's all about you and what makes your soul dance.

And guess what? There's no right or wrong — it's all about progress. Creating a colorful palette of exercises that suit your needs is like designing your very own wellness adventure.

But here's the bonus tip — chat with your healthcare provider or a fitness expert before you dive in. They're like your mentors, helping you fine-tune your plan, ensuring it's tailored to your fitness level and any unique needs.

So, my marvelous friend, let's make your exercise journey an art form. Just like menopause is uniquely yours, your workouts are your own masterpiece. With every step, every move, and every deep breath, you're painting your canvas of well-being with vibrant strokes that light up your journey.

Now, how about energy? It's like your personal fuel for life's adventures. Menopause might throw in a few energy dips, but exercise? It's like your superhero cape, sweeping in and banishing those feelings of sluggishness. When you move, it's like your body's wake-up call — suddenly, you're ready to conquer the day with a spirit that's unstoppable.

But wait, there's more! It's about that sense of empowerment — the feeling that you're the captain of your ship. Exercise is like your compass, guiding you towards accomplishments and achievements. Every step you take, every milestone you reach, it's like a nod from the universe, saying, "You've got this!" It's a reminder that you're capable, strong, and you're writing your own story.

So, how do you elevate your quality of life? It's all about choosing moves that light up your heart. Whether it's a sunrise walk, a dance class that brings out your inner diva, or even a gentle yoga session, the choice is yours. It's not about competition; it's about connection—to your body, to your soul, and to the moments that make life truly worth living. And here's the secret sauce—consistency. Regular exercise is like a promise to yourself. It's like saying, "I'm here for every beautiful moment, every challenge, and every victory." It's a declaration that you're the author of your own story, and it's a celebration of life in all its splendor.

So, my incredible friend, let's step into the spotlight of our own lives. Menopause might be changing the script a little, but you? You're the star, and every move, every choice, and every heartbeat is an invitation to live fully, love deeply, and embrace every moment. Your quality of life is a gift, and with every choice, you're unwrapping it with a heart that's wide open.

Chapter 5: Managing Emotional Wellness

Riding the Emotional Waves - Navigating Mood Swings and More

Let's dive into those mood swings, anxiety, and that emotional roller coaster that menopause might throw your way. Think of this as your emotional toolkit for the journey, a little guide to help you ride those waves and keep your spirit shining through it all.

Mood swings, anxiety, and even that unexpected guest called depression might show up are among the emotional challenges that some women may experience during the menopausal transition. While menopause is a natural phase of life, the hormonal fluctuations that occur can have a significant impact on mental and emotional well-being. Understanding these emotional changes and implementing effective coping strategies can empower women to navigate this phase with resilience and grace.

Mood Swings:

Hey there, soul sister! Let's dig a little deeper into something that might feel like a whirlwind dance of emotions — mood swings. You know, those moments when you go from feeling like a rock star to wondering if you're caught in a storm. Well, guess what? You're not alone, and there's a lot of science and self-care magic that can help you navigate these twists and turns.

Picture this: mood swings are like your emotions doing the cha-cha. Suddenly, you're salsa-ing from joy to frustration, and you might even do a quickstep into anger. It's like your emotional GPS went a little haywire. Those hormones that once were a perfectly choreographed dance team? They're like a jazz band that's playing some unexpected notes. Estrogen and progesterone, those hormonal MVPs, are the ones responsible for this emotional symphony. They're like the conductors of your mood train, sometimes leading you through a symphony and other times through a rock concert.

But here's the science secret — those same hormone changes that can give you hot flashes and night sweats? They're also shaking hands with your brain's neurotransmitters. It's like they're all at a party, and suddenly, your emotions do the Macarena. But fear not, because you're the DJ of your own party, and there are a bunch of tunes you can play to keep the vibes groovy.

Now, here's the self-care magic — it's like your backstage pass to emotional balance. Regular exercise? It's like your daily dose of mood-enhancing vitamins. Mindfulness practices? They're like your mental yoga, keeping your thoughts flexible and your emotions grounded. And oh, stress reduction techniques? They're like your secret weapon against those emotional thunderstorms.

Remember, you're not dancing alone through these mood swings. You've got science, you've got self-care, and you've got an entire tribe of women who are right there on the dance floor with you. So, let's groove through these mood shifts with grace and a touch of your unique style. After all, this menopause journey? It's your very own dance, and those mood swings? They're just a part of the rhythm that makes you beautifully, authentically you.

Anxiety:

Let's jump into something that can feel like a bit of a tango with your thoughts – anxiety. You know, those moments when your mind does a high-speed dance, making your heart skip a beat? Well, I've got a cozy blanket of understanding and some calming techniques to share with you.

Imagine this: anxiety is like your thoughts throwing a party, and suddenly, it feels like the music's turned up a little too loud. Restlessness, unease, and that endless loop of worry? They're like the unexpected guests crashing your gathering. Hormones are like the DJ, and they're experimenting with your brain chemistry, particularly those neurotransmitters — serotonin and dopamine. It's like they're jamming to a different tune, sometimes creating this anxiety-filled remix in your mind.

But here's the secret: life's transitions are like the dance moves you're still learning. Menopause? It's like that whole new routine that you're mastering step by step. And the concerns about aging, the thoughts about the future, they're like dance partners that sometimes lead you astray. It's okay, darling, because you've got the power to lead this dance.

Now, let's talk about self-care that's like a warm hug for your anxious mind. Deep breathing? It's like your secret recipe for a calming cocktail. Progressive muscle relaxation? It's like a soothing massage for your nerves. And yoga? It's like your emotional stretching routine, helping you find that tranquil space within you.

So, here's the truth—you're not alone in this dance with anxiety. Hormones might shake things up, but you've got a repertoire of techniques to help you find your center. Remember, anxiety is just a visitor, and you're the gracious host who knows how to show it to the door. With each deep breath, each moment of mindfulness, you're telling anxiety that it's not the star of the show. You are. And you're dancing through this menopause journey with strength, resilience, and a heart that's ready to find its calm amid the storm.

Depression:

Those moments when the world feels a bit heavy, your energy is a little dimmed, and that spark of joy seems to have taken a vacation. You know what? You're not alone in this, and I'm here to remind you that there's a bright light waiting for you at the end of this tunnel.

Imagine this: depression is like a cloud that's temporarily blocking your sunshine. Feelings of sadness, that sense of being drained, and a lack of interest in things you once loved? They're like unexpected guests who've overstayed their welcome. And hormones? Well, they're like the orchestrators of this emotional symphony. They're waving their batons, sometimes adding a few offbeat notes to your mood.

Here's the science scoop—hormonal changes are like the mood swing in the emotional playground. Estrogen, that superstar hormone, plays a role in serotonin receptors—your brain's mood regulators. When estrogen levels take a dip, it's like those receptors get a little out of tune. But guess what?

You're about to be the conductor of your emotional orchestra, and you've got the power to guide those notes back into harmony.

Now, let's talk about your self-care toolkit—it's like your shield against the clouds. Professional support, like counseling or therapy? It's like your superhero cape, equipping you with the tools to navigate through the shadows. And don't forget about the healing magic of everyday practices. Regular physical activity, those warm connections with friends, and a diet of nutrient-rich foods? They're like rays of light breaking through the gloom.

But here's the truth. Those mood swings, anxiety, and depression? They're not the main characters of your menopause story. You are. And the beauty lies in your power to rewrite the script. With every conversation with your healthcare provider, every hug from a friend, and every step you take towards self-care, you're affirming that this journey is yours to conquer.

So let's hold space for those moments when the clouds gather. But let's also remember that they're just passing through. You're not alone in this. On the other side of those clouds, there's a sky filled with stars—your potential, your dreams, and your resilience. You've got the strength to navigate these emotional currents and to emerge from this transformative phase with grace, wisdom, and an even stronger sense of self.

Finding Inner Peace - Embracing Mindfulness for Emotional Well-being

You know, that magical practice that helps you stay present, even when life throws you a few curveballs? Well, guess what? Mindfulness is your companion for navigating the emotional roller coaster of menopause with a touch of grace and a dash of self-love.

Imagine this: mindfulness is like having your own emotional anchor. It's your secret sauce for keeping your cool when those mood swings and waves of emotions hit. Let's break down some mindfulness moves that you can weave into your daily life:

1. Mindful Breathing: It's like taking a mini-vacation for your mind. Find a cozy corner, take a few deep breaths, and just feel the air flowing in and out. Your breath? It's like the gentle reminder that you're here right now. It's like your mind's personal chill pill, reducing stress and inviting calm.

2. Body Scan Meditation: This one's like a spa day for your soul. Close your eyes, and in your mind, start from your toes and travel all the way up to your head. Notice any little sensations, any tensions — it's like giving your body a hug from the inside. This practice? It's like your permission slip to feel, to let go, and to connect.

3. Mindful Eating: Let's make mealtime a mindful masterpiece. Take a moment to truly taste your food — the flavors, the textures. It's like a date with your plate, a moment to savor and nourish your body. And guess what? This practice is like your secret weapon for building a kinder relationship with food and your own body.

4. Grounding Techniques: When anxiety taps on your door, grounding techniques are like your welcome mat. Look around — name five things you see, four things you touch, three things you hear, two things you smell, and one thing you taste. It's like an instant ticket to the present moment, letting go of those anxious thoughts.

5. Loving-Kindness Meditation: This meditation? It's like a love note to your heart. Sit quietly and let these phrases fill your space: "May I be happy, may I be healthy, may I live with ease." And then, let that warmth extend to others, even to those who might rub you the wrong way. It's like sharing a cup of compassion.

Mindfulness isn't about waving a wand to banish emotions. Nope, it's about inviting them to dance, about holding space for whatever shows up. These practices? They're like your emotional Swiss Army knife. Regular use can lead to a smoother ride on the emotional roller coaster — better emotional balance, a deeper understanding of yourself, and a stronger connection to the present moment.

Mindfulness is your trusty partner. It's your reminder to slow down, breathe, and embrace each moment with a sprinkle of grace and a lot of self-love. Remember, you're not just navigating this phase – you're learning, growing, and embracing the beautiful mess of being human. And with mindfulness as your compass, you will find your way to that sweet spot of inner balance and well-being.

Mindfulness is not about eliminating difficult emotions, but rather developing a compassionate and nonjudgmental awareness of them. Regular practice of these mindfulness techniques can lead to improved emotional regulation, greater self-awareness, and enhanced overall well-being. As you journey through menopause, incorporating mindfulness into your daily routine can be a valuable resource for navigating

emotional challenges with grace and cultivating a deeper
sense of inner balance.

Embracing Support - Seeking Guidance and Counselling through Menopause

You know, those moments when you could use a bit of
guidance, a listening ear, and a helping hand to navigate the
twists and turns? Well, guess what? You're not alone in this,
and reaching out for a bit of expert support is like giving
yourself a big warm hug.

Picture this: seeking professional support is like having a GPS
for your menopause journey. Those twists and turns? They're
the emotional roller coaster that's part of the ride. But having a
healthcare provider or counselor who specializes in women's
health and menopause? It's like having a trusted co-pilot who
knows the terrain like the back of their hand.

1. Expert Guidance: It's like having a compass pointing you in
the right direction. Healthcare providers and therapists who
specialize in menopause are like your personal guides
through this transformative phase. They'll give you the
lowdown on hormonal changes, symptom management, and
all those treatment options. Plus, they'll make sure you're not
missing any vital checkpoints on your journey.

2. Emotional Validation: Menopause is like a swirl of
emotions – mood swings, anxiety, and even a touch of
uncertainty. Imagine having a space where you can just pour
it all out with no judgment. That's what professional
counseling is all about. It's like a cozy corner where you can
express yourself and feel heard and understood.

3. Coping Strategies: Think of therapists as your emotional toolkit creators. They'll equip you with techniques that are like superhero moves against stress and anxiety. Cognitive-behavioral techniques? They're like your mental gymnastics, helping you build resilience. Mindfulness practices? They're like your secret recipe for staying grounded.

4. Relationship Support: Menopause can sometimes toss a few pebbles into your relationship pond. But guess what? Couples counseling is like having a mediator who helps you both navigate those waves. It's like having someone who speaks the language of emotions, helping you and your partner understand each other better.

5. Hormone Therapy Decisions: Thinking about hormone therapy? You're like a detective searching for the best clues. Healthcare providers are your expert investigators, breaking down the pros, cons, and potential side effects of different options. It's like having a decision-making partner who's got your back.

6. Holistic Well-being: Professional support is like your holistic health haven. It's not just about the symptoms—it's about your whole well-being. Discussions about nutrition, exercise, sleep, and stress? They're like pieces of a puzzle that fit together to create your unique menopause journey.

Taking this step? It's like opening a door to a world of understanding, guidance, and empowerment. It's like saying, "Hey, I value my emotional well-being, and I'm strong enough to ask for help when I need it." Whether it's one-on-one chats, group therapy, or medical consultations, seeking professional support is like a treasure trove of insights, tools, and guidance. And remember, dear friend, you're not just navigating menopause—you're sailing through it with a crew of experts who've got your best interests at heart. So go ahead, reach out, and let that expert support be your wind as you navigate this transformative phase with grace, resilience, and a heart full of courage.

Chapter 6: Sleep, Rest, and Energy Renewal

Sweet Dreams - Navigating Sleep Disruptions in Menopause

You know, those nights when your sleep seems to play a game of hide-and-seek? Well, guess what? You're not alone in this sleep adventure, and understanding what's going on can be like having a flashlight to guide you through the dark.

Hormonal Roller Coaster: Imagine your hormones as a bunch of mischievous fairies playing with your sleep patterns. The dip in estrogen levels during menopause can throw your sleep-related hormones, like melatonin and cortisol, into a bit of a dance-off. It's like they're partying when you're trying to snooze, causing you to struggle with falling asleep, staying asleep, or enjoying a deep sleep.

Hot Flashes and Night Sweats: Ever had those moments when your body decides it's time for a surprise heat wave? Hot flashes and night sweats can be like a fire alarm going off in the middle of the night. They wake you up, leave you sweaty and uncomfortable, and even make it a struggle to drift back into slumber. Taming these fiery moments through lifestyle tweaks, relaxation practices, and possibly some medical magic can make your nights cooler and more restful.

Mood Swings and Anxiety: Emotions are like uninvited party crashers sometimes, right? Mood swings and anxiety can be like those noisy guests disrupting your sleep soiree. Racing thoughts, stress, and anxiety can make it tough to wind down and drift into dreamland. But hey, here's the secret pass to better sleep: relaxation practices! Think of them as your VIP ticket to calming the mind and inviting in peaceful sleep.

Bathroom Breaks: Imagine your bladder as a tap that's suddenly decided to stay open all night. Menopause can sometimes lead to more trips to the bathroom than you'd prefer, especially during the night. It's like your sleep's playing a game of tag with your bladder, causing those nighttime wake-up calls. But worry not—finding ways to manage these midnight dashes can restore your uninterrupted sleep.

Sleep Apnea: Ever heard of the snoring monster called sleep apnea? It's like the sneaky culprit that can mess with your sleep. Menopause might increase your chances of encountering this snooze saboteur. Sleep apnea can cause you to wake up suddenly because of pauses in your breathing, throwing your sleep into disarray. Getting a sleep study and any necessary treatment can shoo away this disruptive guest.

Remember, lovely, understanding what's behind those sleep disruptions is like having a secret recipe for sweet slumber. Exploring strategies to manage each factor—from cooling down hot flashes to embracing relaxation practices — can be your roadmap to better sleep. And hey, if you find yourself on a sleepless journey, know that you're not alone. Many women are right there with you, facing the same nighttime adventures.

So, whether you're sipping calming tea before bed, practicing those relaxation tricks, or considering a sleep study, know that you're taking steps toward peaceful nights. Sleep disruptions might be part of the menopause package, but you've got the power to make your nights dreamier. With a mix of understanding, patience, and a dash of sleep wisdom, you're on your way to taming those sleep dragons and embracing the magic of restful slumber once more.

Unleash the Sleep Fairy - Tips for Sweet Slumber during Menopause

Hey there, sleep seeker! Let's dive into the magical world of sleep and discover some tricks to make those Z's a little more accessible. Menopause might have thrown a curveball at your sleep routine, but fear not—we've got a treasure trove of tips to create a sleep haven that even the sleep fairy would envy.

Create a Sleep Oasis: Picture this: your bedroom as a cozy cocoon of tranquility. Keep it cool, dark, and serene. Think comfy pillows, soft sheets, and maybe even a touch of lavender scent to soothe your senses. Adding blackout curtains and a whispering white noise machine can turn your sleep haven into a sanctuary of slumber.

Rise and Shine, Even on weekends: Imagine your body as a clock that loves routine. Going to bed and waking up at the same time every day, even on weekends, helps keep your body's internal clock in check. It's like having a daily rendezvous with sleep.

The Digital Detour: Ever noticed how screens can be like little sleep stealers? Avoid those electronic gadgets at least an hour before bedtime. Their blue light can mess with your melatonin production, making it harder to fall asleep. Why not replace screen time with a cozy book or a cup of herbal tea?

Nibble Wisely: That bedtime snack—it matters! Skip the heavy meals, caffeine, and cocktails close to bedtime. Your digestive system will thank you, and your sleep will be less likely to play hide-and-seek.

Exercise, but Not Too Late: You know that energizing exercise routine? It's like a superhero for sleep—but only if you time it right. Engage in regular physical activity, but let's avoid the high-energy workouts right before bed. That way, you're not inviting Mr. Wide Awake to your slumber party.

Let Stress Take a Hike: Stress is like an unwelcome party crasher at bedtime. Give it the boot by practicing relaxation techniques. Deep breaths, calming meditations, and maybe even a warm bath can usher in tranquility and prepare you for a date with sweet dreams.

Hydrate Early: Picture your bladder as a bedtime bouncer. To minimize those nighttime trips to the bathroom, cut down on fluids in the evening. That way, your sleep won't get interrupted by midnight pit stops.

When in Doubt, Seek Help: You're not alone in this sleep adventure. If sleep disruptions are overstaying their welcome, consider chatting with a healthcare provider. They're like sleep detectives who can offer insights, suggest sleep studies if needed, and explore options to bring back those dreamy nights.

Remember, lovely, these tips are like puzzle pieces that can fit into your unique sleep routine. Menopause might have shaken things up, but you're the conductor of your sleep symphony. With a bit of mindful tinkering, your sleep oasis can become a reality. Sweet dreams are just around the corner, and you've got the power to welcome them with open arms.

So, dim the lights, turn off those screens, and cozy up for a sleep journey that's worthy of a fairy tale.

Crafting Your Sleep Sanctuary - A Haven for Dreamy Nights

Hey there, sleep enthusiast! Let's dive into the wonderful world of sleep sanctuaries and unravel the secrets to crafting the ultimate cozy cocoon for those precious Z's. Menopause might have stirred the sleep pot a bit, but fear not—we're here to sprinkle some magic and create a sleep environment that'll have you snoozing like a pro.

The Bed of Dreams: Picture this—your bed as a cloud of comfort waiting to whisk you away. A mattress that's just right for you, accompanied by soft, breathable sheets and pillows, is the recipe for a sleep haven. Oh, and let's not forget those temperature-regulating materials to tackle those pesky night sweats.

Lights, But Make Them Dim: Imagine your bedroom basking in the warm glow of soft, dim lights. Bid farewell to those harsh, bright lights that can mess with your sleep hormone production. Let's coax your body into relaxation mode with gentle, calming lighting.

Declutter for Zen Vibes: Ever heard of a clutter-free mind? Well, a clutter-free bedroom comes close! Organize your space, keep it tidy, and bid adieu to visual distractions. A serene room equals a serene mind ready for dreamland adventures.

Colors of Calm: Think peaceful, soothing colors for your sleep sanctuary. Imagine soft blues, gentle greens, and neutral tones enveloping you in tranquility. Say no to the bold and the bright – we're aiming for serenity, not stimulation.

White Noise Magic: Enter white noise machines and fans, your secret weapons against disruptive sounds. They create a soothing auditory backdrop that's perfect for a peaceful sleep symphony. You can also opt for nature's lullabies – think raindrops or ocean waves.

Thermostat Harmony: Goldilocks would approve – not too hot, not too cold, just right. A cozy room temperature, usually on the cooler side, helps set the stage for dreamy slumber. And guess what? Breathable bedding materials can keep your temperature in check.

Aromatherapy Elegance: Let's introduce the magic of aromatherapy. Lavender, chamomile, vanilla – these scents are like a lullaby for your senses. Try essential oils, room sprays, or scented candles to create an atmosphere of serenity.

Decor for Zen: Surround yourself with decor that whispers relaxation. Pictures that make you smile, artwork that soothes your soul – they all have a place in your sleep sanctuary. Let your surroundings carry you to dreamland on a cloud of calm.

Gadget-Free Zone: Let's give your gadgets a vacation. Remove those electronic devices from your sleep space. The blue light they emit can mess with your sleep hormone, so it's best to leave them out of your slumber party.

By crafting a sleep sanctuary tailored to your preferences, you're inviting restful nights and rejuvenating slumber into your life. Remember, lovely, this is your personal haven, and you hold the magic wand. Sweet dreams are just a cozy sleep environment away, and with a sprinkle of care and creativity, you're well on your way to transforming your nights into a dreamy adventure. So, dim the lights, fluff those pillows, and drift off into a world of tranquil sleep.

Nurturing Your Sleep Naturally - A Guide to Menopause Sleep Harmony

Hey there, sleep explorer! Let's venture into the world of natural remedies and sleep hygiene, your trusty companions on the quest for peaceful slumber. Menopause might throw some curveballs your way, but fear not—we've got a toolkit of holistic approaches to help you sail smoothly through those sleep disruptions.

The Magic of Nature's Elixirs:

1. Herbal Tea Magic: Imagine winding down with a cup of chamomile, valerian root, or passionflower tea. These herbal heroes have been soothing souls for ages, promoting relaxation and better sleep. Sip on these comforting concoctions as part of your bedtime ritual.

2. Aromatherapy Oasis: Say hello to essential oils—your aromatic allies for better sleep. Lavender, bergamot, cedar wood—they're like a fragrant lullaby for your senses. Diffuse them or add a few drops to your bath to create a dreamy atmosphere.

3. Magnesium Marvel: Meet magnesium, your relaxation sidekick. It helps muscles unwind and regulate melatonin—

your sleep hormone. Nosh on magnesium-rich foods like leafy greens, nuts, and seeds, or consider a supplement under the guidance of a healthcare pro.

4. Melatonin Magic: Say hi to melatonin — your sleep-wake cycle superhero. Melatonin supplements, in the right dose and with guidance, and I can't stress that enough as typically the doses are too high, can help reset your internal clock for dreamier nights.

Embracing the Art of Sleep Hygiene:

1. Schedule Love: Imagine having a sleep rendezvous with your bed at the same time every day. This consistency is your sleep BFF, helping your internal clock find its groove.

2. Screen Detox: Give your screens a break before bedtime. The blue light they emit can mess with your melatonin production. Instead, opt for a calming pre-sleep ritual, like reading or gentle stretching.

3. Bedroom Zen Zone: Transform your sleep space into a relaxation oasis. Ditch the work, the TV, and those electronic devices. Let your bedroom be a haven for slumber and serenity.

4. Caffeine Cut-off: Skip the caffeine and nicotine party before bedtime. They're sleep disruptors, and we're all about cozy slumber soirées.

5. Movement Matters: Get your groove on with regular physical activity, but avoid intense workouts close to bedtime. Exercise is a sleep champion, but it's better than a daytime dance partner.

6. Relaxation Rituals: Imagine unwinding with deep breaths, muscle relaxation, or meditation. These relaxation rendezvous can soothe your mind and guide you into the land of dreams.

7. Light Love: Soak up the sun during the day to keep your internal clock ticking. But when it's time to wind down, dim those lights and set the stage for tranquil sleep.

8. Fluid Finesse: Sip smartly by reducing your fluid intake before bedtime. No need for those midnight bathroom breaks to crash your sleep party.

9. Cozy Cocoon: Think of your bed as your cloud of comfort. Invest in a comfortable mattress, soft pillows, and breathable bedding. Create a haven that's cool, dark, and ready for your dreams.

By embracing natural remedies and weaving sleep hygiene into your routine, you're crafting a roadmap to dreamland that's uniquely yours. Remember, lovely, these are tools in your sleep treasure chest—ones you can tailor to your taste. Let's reclaim your nights, nurture your sleep, and navigate the menopause journey with the grace of a sleep champion. Sweet dreams await, and with a dash of nature's magic and some sleep-friendly practices, you're well on your way to snuggling up with slumber once again.

Chapter 7: Natural Approaches to Symptom Relief

Navigating Nature's Aids - A Guide to Herbal Remedies and Supplements for Menopause

If you're exploring the realm of herbal remedies and supplements for those menopause moments, you're not alone. For centuries, women have turned to nature's treasures to find relief and support during this transformative phase. But, as with any adventure, a little guidance is essential. Before diving in, let's chat about how to approach these remedies with wisdom and care.

Unveiling Nature's Secrets:

1. Black Cohosh: Ah, the legend of black cohosh! This herbal wizard is renowned for its power against hot flashes and night sweats. It's like having a secret weapon that mimics estrogen's effects. But remember, it's like a magic potion that works differently for each of us, and we're still uncovering its long-term story.

2. Dong Quai: Imagine a cup of tea with a hint of Dong Quai – an ancient Chinese herb for harmonizing hormones. It's whispered to ease hot flashes, mood swings, and even that pesky vaginal dryness. But, here's the deal: consult your healthcare oracle before sipping, especially if blood clotting's been a nemesis.

3. Red Clover: Enter the realm of red clover — home to phytoestrogens, those clever plant compounds that mimic estrogen. They're like nature's version of backup dancers, soothing hot flashes and seeking hormonal balance. But remember, this story is still unfolding, and more research scrolls are needed.

4. Evening Primrose: Picture this: evening primrose oil, a potion with gamma-linolenic acid (GLA), dancing to ease breast tenderness and mood swings. It's like a serene symphony for your senses, but the research notes are in early drafts, so don't forget your healthcare maestro's counsel.

5. Flaxseed: Imagine flaxseed — a gift packed with omega-3s and lignans, nature's subtle mimicry of estrogen. It's like a plant-powered hug, embracing hot flashes and heart health. While the whispers of studies suggest benefits, keep in mind that research chapters are still being penned.

6. Vitamin D: Meet vitamin D — your bone's BFF and a ray of sunshine for mood swings and immune strength. You can find it in sunlit paths or foods like fish, but sometimes, a supplement sidekick is just what the healthcare scroll ordered.

7. Calcium and Magnesium: Think of calcium and magnesium as the dynamic duo for bones and relaxation. These trusty minerals ease muscle cramps and dance to promote well-being. They're like the guardians of your fortress, but don't forget, sometimes, a supplement can be the extra armor you need.

Nurturing Nature's Gifts with Care:

Before you set sail on your herbal journey, pause for a heart-to-heart with your healthcare guardian. Their wisdom is your compass through uncharted waters. They'll help you decipher which herbal allies are safe for your unique tale, and if any potential interactions are lurking. While natural approaches can provide relief for some women, it's crucial to prioritize safety and seek professional guidance to ensure that your chosen remedies are appropriate and effective for your needs.

While herbal remedies and supplements can be companions along the way, they're part of a greater story. Keep your healthcare sage close by and let them guide you to the chapters that align with your needs. Embrace these natural allies, but with the armor of caution and the wisdom of counsel. Together, you're crafting a narrative of well-being and care, one herb at a time.

Scented Serenity - Embracing Essential Oils and Aromatherapy for Relaxation

Let's talk about diving into the world of aromatherapy and essential oils—a journey that's all about surrounding yourself with scents that feel like a warm hug for your senses. Imagine soothing aromas filling the air, like whispered secrets of ancient remedies that can ease your stress and wrap you in a cozy cocoon of relaxation.

A Symphony for Your Senses:

Think of aromatherapy as a sensory symphony — a melody of essential oils that plays a tune that resonates deep within you. As you inhale these scents, they waltz their way to a special place in your brain called the limbic system. It's the cozy corner where your emotions, memories, and stress responses have heart-to-heart conversations.

By tapping into this magical connection, aromatherapy orchestrates a sense of calmness and balance. Imagine it as a conductor, guiding your emotions into a harmonious rhythm. For those moments when anxiety knocks on your door, or mood swings try to steal the spotlight, aromatherapy steps in with a peaceful encore.

Your Relaxation Dream Team:

Let's meet some of the superstar oils that play a leading role in relaxation:

1. Lavender: it's like a bouquet of serenity. With its gentle, floral notes, it's the go-to essential oil for relaxation. Imagine a warm bath infused with lavender, or a few drops on your pillow, casting a spell of calmness and improved sleep quality.

2. Chamomile: Enter chamomile — your cozy cup of tea transformed into an aromatic remedy. Whether it's Roman or German chamomile, this essential oil wraps you in a calming embrace, chasing away anxiety and restlessness.

3. Ylang Ylang: Say hello to ylang ylang — an exotic dancer of the essential oil world. Its sweet aroma dances in the air, creating a tranquil ambiance that helps lower blood pressure, ease stress, and invite relaxation.

4. Bergamot: the citrusy sunrise that brightens your mood. Picture its uplifting scent melting away tension and anxiety, leaving you with a refreshed spirit and a positive outlook.

5. Frankincense: the wise elder of essential oils. Its warm and woody aroma is like a hug from within, grounding you in moments of meditation and mindfulness.

A Whiff of Wisdom:

Now, here's the secret sauce — before you dive into this fragrant journey, have a chat with your healthcare confidant. Essential oils are powerful allies, but even powerful allies need a little guidance. Consult your healthcare fairy godmother to ensure that the scents you choose align with your wellness path.

Picture aromatherapy as a gentle breeze, soothing your spirit and guiding you toward relaxation. Allow these essences to weave their magic as you create your sanctuary of serenity. Whether it's a calming bath, a diffuser dancing with scent, or a gentle massage, let these aromatic companions embrace you with their natural wonders.

Embracing the Aroma Adventure - Weaving Aromatherapy into Your Everyday

If you're ready to embark on a fragrant journey that'll make your senses sing, then let's dive into the world of aromatherapy together. It's like stepping into a garden of scents that can whisk you away to a world of relaxation and calm.

Scented Symphony:

Imagine your home as a symphony hall, and essential oils are the musicians playing a soothing melody that resonates with your soul. These little aromatic powerhouses can transform any space into a tranquil sanctuary — a place where stress meets its match and relaxation takes center stage.

Scent in the Air:

Here's how you can sprinkle a little aroma magic into your daily routine:

1. Dance of the Diffusers: Essential oil diffusers are your new BFFs. These nifty gadgets sprinkle droplets of enchanting scent into the air, turning your room into a haven of calm. Set one up in your bedroom or living room and let the aroma weave its charm.

2. Sensational Soaks: Ah, the aromatic bath — a lavish escape from the hustle and bustle. A few drops of your favorite essential oil in a warm bath, and suddenly you're surrounded by a fragrant embrace. Picture yourself soaking in a tub of relaxation, letting the day's worries melt away.

3. Massage Magic: Ready for some self-pampering? Dilute a drop or two of essential oil with a carrier oil (like jojoba or coconut oil) and treat yourself to a gentle massage. It's like a soothing spa day, right in the comfort of your own space.

4. Inhale, Exhale: Inhaling the goodness of essential oils directly from the bottle can be an instant mood-lifter. Need a pick-me-up during the day? A quick whiff can transport you to a fragrant paradise.

The Safety Dance:

Now, before we get too carried away in this aromatic symphony, let's have a chat about safety. Just like you'd consult a trusted friend for advice, it's a good idea to have a heart-to-heart with your healthcare provider before you dive into essential oils. They can give you the green light and ensure that your wellness journey is smooth sailing.

Quality matters too! Choose pure, high-quality essential oils to get the best experience. And don't forget, a little goes a long way. Always follow the recommended guidelines for safe usage and dilution. We want to wrap you in relaxation, not skin irritations.

So, dear aroma explorer, by infusing aromatherapy into your routine, you're gifting yourself moments of tranquility and serenity. You're creating a personal haven of relaxation amidst the hustle and bustle of life. So, go ahead, let the scents whisk you away, and let your senses dance to the rhythm of calmness during your menopausal journey.

Zen Vibes and Ancient Wisdom - Acupuncture and Yoga as Menopause Allies

If you're seeking holistic ways to embrace your menopause journey, let's delve into two powerful alternatives that have been making waves in the wellness world: acupuncture and yoga. Picture this as your passport to a serene state of mind and body.

Needles of Harmony: Acupuncture

Imagine a delicate dance of needles that helps your body find its equilibrium—that's acupuncture! This ancient practice, rooted in Chinese healing wisdom, involves the gentle insertion of ultra-fine needles into specific points on your body. It's like giving your body a gentle nudge to get back into its natural rhythm.

Acupuncture during menopause? You bet! This needle magic can target those pesky hot flashes, ease sleep disruptions, and tame mood swings. How? By encouraging the release of calming hormones and neurotransmitters. It's like a secret code that whispers to your body, "Relax, we got this." Many women swear by its calming effects and the soothing sense of relief it brings.

Embrace the Mat: Yoga

Now, let's talk yoga—your inner calm's best friend. Yoga is like a symphony of movement, breath, and mindfulness that serenades your body and mind. Those beautiful poses? They're not just about flexibility; they're about balance and strength—things we all need during menopause.

You know those hot flashes that sometimes take center stage? Yoga can be your backstage pass to soothing them. It helps

you embrace sleep with open arms, melts away stress, and
even gives your emotional well-being a boost. It's like a warm,
comforting hug that whispers, "You're doing great, and you're
strong."

Exploring Your Path:

Remember, your journey is unique, just like you. While
acupuncture and yoga are wonderful companions, always
consult your healthcare provider before embarking on any
new adventure. And if you decide to hop on the acupuncture
table or the yoga mat, choose professionals who understand
your menopause journey.

You're crafting your path to balance and well-being, and these
alternatives are here to join you on the ride. Whether it's the
delicate touch of acupuncture or the serene flow of yoga,
know that you're nurturing your body and mind with ancient
wisdom and modern harmony. So go ahead, step into your
Zen zone and let your menopause journey become a beautiful
tapestry of tranquility and strength.

Wholehearted Wellness - Tailoring
Acupuncture and Yoga to Your Journey:

Wholeness in Harmony: Holistic Approach

Imagine your body as a symphony, where each note is
connected to the next—that's what acupuncture and yoga are

all about! They don't just focus on isolated symptoms; they see you as the masterpiece you are, woven together with threads of emotion, spirit, and body. They get it—it's not just about the hot flashes; it's about taming stress, finding peace, and nurturing your essence.

Your Journey, Your Way: Individualization

Guess what? These practices are like tailor-made outfits for your well-being. Acupuncture is all about pinpointing the spots that need a little extra love—whether it's those mood swings or sleep troubles. It's like giving your body a custom hug, soothing exactly where it needs it.

Now, picture yoga as your personal dance—one that respects where you are on your journey. No need to twist yourself into a pretzel (unless you want to!). Yoga meets you where you are, honoring your fitness level and preferences. It's like a supportive friend saying, "Let's move, breathe, and find peace — your way."

Your Journey, Your Tempo:

What works for one might not work for another, and that's perfectly okay. These practices are like a buffet of well-being; you get to choose what resonates with you. And remember, it's your journey—embrace it, tweak it, and make it yours.

When you venture into the world of acupuncture and yoga, it's like stepping onto sacred ground. You're in safe hands with certified experts who understand the uniqueness of your menopause journey. They're your guides to the symphony of well-being, crafting sessions that soothe, support, and empower.

So, let these practices blend seamlessly into your life, reminding you that your well-being matters — body, mind, and spirit. With acupuncture's pinpointed care and yoga's gentle embrace, you're on a path to wholehearted wellness. Get ready to write your well-being story, one holistic chapter at a time.

Chapter 8: Navigating Intimate Health

Embracing Intimate Changes - Navigating Libido and Vaginal Health in Menopause

Hey there, fabulous soul! Ready to dive into a topic that's as intimate as sharing secrets with your best friend? Buckle up, we are about to explore the world of libido and vaginal health during the menopause journey—no taboos, just real talk.

The Hormonal Tango: Changes in Libido

Picture this: hormones dancing like stars in the night sky, shaping your emotions, body, and, yes, your libido. During menopause, these hormones do the cha-cha, and it's perfectly normal for your libido to swing with them. Those mood swings and fatigue aren't just playing a solo; they're part of this dance too.

Now, when the curtains come down and it's time for a romantic evening, your libido might not show up as often as before. And that's okay, darling! It's not just hormones; life's little stresses and changes can grab the spotlight too. And remember, that's totally normal.

The Vagina Chronicles: Vaginal Health Changes

Let's talk about your intimate space – the vagina. Estrogen, your body's VIP, keeps things comfortable and thriving down there. But during menopause, it's like estrogen took a vacation, and your vaginal lining might be less plump and more delicate.

Ever heard of "vaginal atrophy"? Think of it as the unwelcome guest at your body's party. As estrogen levels drop, it can lead to dryness, itching, and a burning sensation. And yes, that's not all—it can make intimacy a bit, well, uncomfortable. Your vagina's pH balance might also be all over the place, leaving you more prone to infections.

No Shame, Just Understanding

Changes in libido and vaginal health are like little postcards from menopause, telling you that your body is on a new adventure. Your emotions, desires, and needs matter, and it's time to give them the attention they deserve.

But guess what? You've got this! The beauty of it all is that there are ways to navigate these changes with grace and self-love. From embracing open conversations with your partner to exploring treatments that soothe your intimate spaces, you've got a toolkit at your fingertips.

So, let's dive into this chapter together — no judgment, just understanding. We're tackling the changes in libido and vaginal health head-on, with the power of knowledge and self-care by our side. Get ready to own your journey, embrace the changes, and step into a more intimate and confident you.

Navigating Changes in Libido and Vaginal Health: Your Ultimate Guide

Alright, gorgeous, let's talk about something that's as personal as picking out the perfect lipstick shade—managing changes in libido and vaginal health. No need to blush—we're diving in headfirst and exploring ways to keep the sparks alive during the menopausal ride.

1. Opening Up: The Power of Communication

Picture this: you and your partner sitting down, sharing a cup of tea, and opening up about how you're feeling. Yep, that's the secret sauce—open and honest communication. If you're noticing changes in your libido or the way you experience pleasure, your partner needs to know. Trust me, beautiful, they're not mind-readers. So, chat it out, share your thoughts, concerns, and let your hearts connect on a deeper level.

2. Lifestyle Lovin': Fueling Your Fire

Let's talk self-care, shall we? Engaging in regular physical activity isn't just for those cute workout outfits—it can boost your overall well-being, including your sexual health. Stress, oh stress, it can be a mood-killer. But guess what? Finding ways to manage it—like through yoga, meditation, or simply taking time for yourself — can make a world of difference in how you feel between the sheets. And yes, a balanced diet isn't just about those leafy greens — it's about nourishing your body and keeping that energy high.

3. Set the Stage: Foreplay and Lubrication

Now, let's talk about the art of setting the stage for pleasure. Foreplay isn't just a warm-up; it's a crucial part of the journey. Taking your time, exploring each other's bodies, and allowing that desire to build can make a world of difference. And speaking of comfort, say hello to water-based lubricants. These little wonders can be a game-changer if you're experiencing vaginal dryness. No more discomfort — just smooth sailing.

4. Vaginal TLC: Moisturize and Shine

Remember that feeling of your skin soaking up moisturizer after a shower? Well, your vagina deserves some TLC too. Non-prescription vaginal moisturizers are your new best friends. They'll help keep things comfortable, moist, and happy down there. It's all about taking care of yourself — every inch.

5. The Hormone Chat: Therapy and Support

Hormone therapy, or HRT, might be a topic that pops up. If vaginal atrophy is cramping your style, HRT or localized estrogen therapy might be on the table. Remember, gorgeous, it's a personal choice and something to discuss with your healthcare provider. They'll walk you through the benefits and potential risks, and you get to decide what feels right for you.

6. Flex Those Muscles: Pelvic Floor Exercises

Kegels—they're not just for when you're stuck in traffic. These little exercises can strengthen your pelvic floor muscles, support bladder control, and even enhance your intimate experiences. Who knew flexing could be so fun?

7. Unleash the Pleasure: Sexual Wellness Products

Ready for a little adventure? Some women swear by sexual wellness products. From vibrators to vaginal dilators, these tools are designed to enhance pleasure and make you feel amazing. It's all about embracing what brings you joy and comfort.

8. The Expert Opinion: Seeking Professional Help

When in doubt, reach out. Whether it's your healthcare provider or a specialist in sexual medicine, seeking professional help is a superpower. They've got the knowledge and expertise to guide you through these changes, offering personalized solutions tailored to you.

Beautiful, remember this journey is all about you—your needs, your desires, and your comfort. Embrace it with patience, self-love, and a sprinkle of adventure. From heart-to-heart talks with your partner to trying out new things, you've got a toolkit full of strategies to keep the flames alive. So, go on and explore, gorgeous—your body, your rules.

Navigating Menopause with Your Partner: Building Deeper Bonds

We've talked about changes in libido and vaginal health, but guess what? Your partner is right there with you on this journey. Let's dive into how open communication and maintaining a strong connection can make all the difference as you both navigate the twists and turns of menopause together.

1. Heart-to-Heart Talks: The Power of Honesty

You know those late-night talks over a cup of tea? They're golden. Menopause isn't a secret mission — it's a natural part of life. So, let your partner in on your experiences, fears, and needs. Create a judgment-free zone where you can both share openly. This is a two-way street, darling. Encourage your partner to share too — understanding goes both ways.

2. Learning as a Team: Education is Empowerment

Time for some teamwork! Dive into the world of menopause together. From flipping through informative books to watching videos, the more you both know, the stronger your united front becomes. Doctor's appointments? Attend them together. Knowledge is power, and shared knowledge is unity.

3. Ride the Emotional Rollercoaster — Together

Menopause isn't just about the physical stuff; those mood swings and emotional rollercoasters are part of the package too. Remember, those hormonal shifts aren't a verdict about your relationship. Share how you're feeling and give your partner a peek into your emotional world. Together, you can navigate this bumpy ride and be each other's anchors.

4. Teamwork in the Bedroom: Adapting to Change

Let's talk about the bedroom, shall we? If changes in libido or physical comfort are on the table, speak up, gorgeous. Discuss what feels good, what needs adjusting, and explore new avenues of pleasure. Remember, intimacy isn't just about the physical — emotional closeness matters just as much.

5. New Adventures, New Bonds

Menopause can be a gateway to new beginnings. Think of it as an opportunity to explore new activities together. From hiking trails to art classes, finding shared interests outside of the bedroom can spice up your connection and give you fresh experiences to savor together.

6. Patience is the Secret Ingredient

Patience, my friend, is a superpower. Menopause isn't a race; it's a journey. Support each other through the highs and lows, offering a shoulder during moments of frustration and uncertainty. Remember, your partner's experience is unique, just like yours. Walk the path together with kindness and understanding.

7. When in Doubt, Seek Help Together

If the road gets bumpy and the lines of communication get tangled, don't hesitate to reach out for help. Couples' therapy or counseling can provide a safe space to untangle knots, learn better ways to communicate, and navigate challenges as a united front.

Through thick and thin, open hearts and supportive shoulders, you and your partner can face menopause head-on. It's about weaving your lives together, adapting to change, and emerging with a bond that's unbreakable. So, hold hands, beautiful—this chapter of your journey is one you'll write together.

Embracing Intimate Health as a Single Woman: Your Journey, Your Way

Hey there, fabulous single lady! Menopause isn't just a chapter for couples; it's a journey that's uniquely yours. Let's chat about how you can navigate changes in libido and vaginal health as a single woman and take charge of your intimate well-being.

1. Self-Care and Self-Exploration: Your Body, Your Rules

Guess what? Your body, your rules! Self-care is your secret weapon. Get to know yourself intimately—what makes you tick, what brings you pleasure, and what makes you feel amazing. It's all about tuning into your body's rhythm and discovering what ignites your spark.

2. Open Conversations with Friends: Sharing is Caring

Your friends? They're your rock. Open conversations about menopause can be empowering and reassuring. Share your experiences, swap tips, and let each other know that you're not alone on this journey. And who knows? Your BFF might have a genius solution you hadn't thought of!

3. Professional Guidance: Experts on Your Team

Who says you can't have experts in your corner? If you're experiencing any discomfort or changes that concern you, consider reaching out to a healthcare provider. They're your go-to source for information, guidance, and potential solutions to make sure you're feeling your best.

4. Exploring Sensuality: Taking Charge of Pleasure

Single doesn't mean you can't explore sensuality. Embrace pleasure, whether through self-pleasure or diving into new experiences. There are no boundaries to how you can explore and nourish your own desires.

5. Mindfulness and Self-Love: Nurturing Your Well-Being

Girl, you're a star — treat yourself like one! Practice mindfulness, indulge in self-love, and let go of any judgments or worries. Taking care of your overall well-being can create a positive ripple effect on your intimate health.

6. Staying Informed: Knowledge is Empowerment

Knowledge is your superpower. Stay informed about the changes your body might go through during menopause. The more you understand, the more confident you can navigate this journey.

7. Future Relationships: You, Your Needs, Your Desires

Thinking about future relationships? Remember, you deserve someone who cherishes every aspect of you — including this chapter of your journey. Open communication with a potential partner about your experiences and desires can create a foundation of trust and understanding.

8. Embracing You: Your Journey, Your Way

Ultimately, this journey is all about you. Embrace your uniqueness, your desires, and your path. Whether you're single, dating, or anywhere in between, your intimate health is part of your holistic well-being. Celebrate yourself — you're living life on your terms.
So, single lady, here's to embracing intimate health as a solo superstar. Your journey is an opportunity to explore, discover, and cherish yourself. Own it, embrace it, and let your light shine brightly.

Chapter 9: Empowerment and Self-Care Practices

Self-Compassion: Your Inner Cheerleader

Ever had that inner critic chime in with not-so-nice thoughts? Time to introduce it to your new BFF: self-compassion. Imagine talking to yourself with the warmth and encouragement you'd offer a dear friend. That's self-compassion, and it's a game-changer during menopause.

When those mood swings or moments of self-doubt hit, give yourself a break. You're navigating uncharted waters, and you're doing it with grace. Self-compassion is about acknowledging your challenges without judgment, embracing your feelings, and reminding yourself that you're doing your best.

Two Peas in a Pod: Self-Care and Self-Compassion

Guess what? These two are the dynamic duo of well-being. Self-care is the action—it's saying, "Hey body, I've got your back!" And self-compassion is the inner voice saying, "You're doing great, and you're enough." They're a tag team, each making the other stronger.

As you take those self-care steps, let self-compassion be your co-pilot. If you miss a workout or have a rough day, instead of getting down on yourself, offer a little self-compassion. Treat yourself like you would a close friend — with understanding, kindness, and a sprinkle of encouragement.

Empowerment: Your Menopause Magic

Here's the beautiful part: self-care and self-compassion aren't just practices — they're superpowers. When you blend them, you're arming yourself with a shield of well-being that's tailor made for menopause. You're creating a sacred space where you thrive, embracing the journey with a sense of empowerment and self-assuredness.

As you journey through menopause, let self-care be your love letter to yourself. Let self-compassion be your inner cheerleader. Together, they're your keys to resilience, self-assurance, and a menopausal experience that radiates with well-being and self-love. You've got this!

Setting Boundaries and Prioritizing Your Needs during Menopause

Menopause is like embarking on a personal journey filled with twists and turns. Amidst all the changes, there's something magical about setting boundaries and making yourself a priority. Let's dive into why these practices are like gold nuggets in your treasure chest of well-being.

Embracing Your Needs: It's Your Time

Menopause isn't just a phase; it's a spotlight on your needs.
From the physical shifts, like hot flashes, to the emotional
rollercoaster of mood swings, this is the moment to recognize
what you truly require. It's like giving yourself permission to
say, "Hey, I matter!" It's about tuning in to your body's
whispers and choosing to honor them.

Building Boundaries: Your Energy Fortress

Picture your boundaries as a beautiful garden fence — strong,
yet inviting. In a world buzzing with demands and changes,
boundaries are your secret weapon. They're your way of
saying, "I'm taking care of me." It might set limits on your
time, letting loved ones know when you need space, or
carving out moments just for yourself. These boundaries are
the gatekeepers of your energy, ensuring it's used wisely and
not depleted.

Saying Yes to Self-Care: Your Menopause Supercharge

Self-care isn't selfish; it's a lifeline to your well-being.
Prioritizing self-care during menopause is like giving yourself
a warm hug. It's waking up and saying, "I'm worth it." It
might be that morning yoga session that starts your day with
a smile, savoring a cup of herbal tea, or simply indulging in

moments of solitude. When you show up for yourself, you're
supercharging your resilience, stepping through menopause
with grace, and embracing each change as a testament to your
strength.

You, Unveiled: A Journey to Empowerment

As you embrace boundaries and prioritize self-care, you're
unfurling your wings of empowerment. You're not just
navigating menopause; you're crafting a symphony of well-
being. Think of boundaries as the canvas on which you paint
your self-respect and self-care as the melody that uplifts your
spirit.

Remember that setting boundaries and prioritizing your needs
are your companions on this adventure. They're your way of
saying, "I'm here, and I matter." Let your needs guide you, let
boundaries protect you, and let self-care fuel your radiance.
It's your time to shine!

Benefits of Boundaries and Self-Prioritization:

Hey there, radiant soul! Let's talk about how your
superpowers — setting boundaries and putting yourself first —
are the secret ingredients to turning your menopause journey
into a beautiful adventure.

Welcoming Serenity: Stress Reduction at its Best

Imagine walking through life without carrying the weight of the world on your shoulders. That's what boundaries do — they become your invisible shield against overwhelm. When you say "no" to what drains you and "yes" to what lights you up, you're creating a space for tranquility to flourish. Boundaries are like the gentle breeze that whispers, "You've got this, sister." They let you embrace menopause at your pace, free from the chaos of excessive commitments.

The Dance of Self-Respect: A Symphony of Confidence

Picture yourself in a world where your needs take center stage. That's the power of prioritizing yourself. When you choose self-care, it's like standing up and applauding your own worth. The world sees how you treat yourself, and that radiates into the universe. As you value your well-being, your self-esteem and confidence soar to new heights. It's like wearing a shimmering cloak of self-respect, one that you've crafted with love.

Harmonious Connections: The Joy of Healthy Relationships

Boundaries aren't walls; they're bridges that lead to better relationships. When you communicate your needs clearly, you're allowing your loved ones to understand and respect your journey. It's like giving them a map of your heart, guiding them towards understanding you better. And when they see how you honor your own needs, it inspires a ripple effect. Suddenly, your relationships become gardens of mutual respect and love.

Emotional Serenity: Navigating the Waves

Menopause brings tides of emotions — some high and exhilarating, others low and challenging. That's where self-care steps in, like a lighthouse guiding you through the storm. When you prioritize yourself, you're offering yourself a cushion of emotional resilience. Those mood swings? They're not as daunting. The stresses? They become stepping stones towards growth. Self-prioritization is your toolkit for emotional balance, making you a skilled navigator of your own emotions.

You, the Captain of Empowerment: Steering Your Ship

Boundaries and self-prioritization aren't just practices; they're the wind in your sails, propelling you forward. They give you the power to shape your menopause journey according to your terms. When you set boundaries, you're declaring, "I'm in control of my choices." And when you prioritize yourself, you're saying, "I deserve happiness and well-being." It's like holding the helm of your ship, confidently charting your course through the waves of change.

Remember that setting boundaries and placing yourself at the center of your journey are like sprinkling stardust on your menopause adventure. Embrace the tranquility they offer, adorn yourself in the cloak of self-respect, nurture the gardens of your relationships, and sail through the emotional tides with grace. You're the author of your menopause tale, and these are the chapters that infuse it with magic, resilience, and a whole lot of you!

The Canvas of Renewal: Embrace Change with Open Arms

Imagine your life as a canvas, and menopause as the vibrant strokes of change splashed across it. It's not about erasing what was; it's about adding new hues that bring your story to life. Exploring fresh interests isn't just about filling your time; it's about embracing renewal. It's about saying, "Hey world, I'm evolving, and I'm ready to paint my life with vibrant shades of joy!" So, let's embark on this colorful adventure together.

Creative Whispers of the Soul: Express and Elevate

Have you ever had an urge to dance like nobody's watching or create art that speaks your heart's language? That's your creative spirit calling out during menopause. Engaging in creative pursuits—whether it's crafting, journaling, photography, or playing a musical instrument — gives your inner thoughts a chance to whisper, shout, and echo through your chosen medium. It's like hearing your heart's melody played out in the notes of your passions. Through creative expression, you honor your journey and empower yourself to embrace change with grace.

Confidence: Your Wings to Fly in Uncharted Territories

Stepping into new passions might seem daunting, but trust me, it's your confidence booster in disguise. That feeling of accomplishment when you try something new — that's the secret sauce. Think about it — when you conquer a new challenge, you're telling yourself, "Look what I can do!" This newfound self-assuredness transcends your endeavors, shaping your outlook on life. Suddenly, the menopausal whirlwind becomes an exciting dance of change, and you? You're leading the way with confidence.

Connection: Friends Anew on the Horizon

Remember when you joined clubs in school and made friends who shared your interests? Guess what? Menopause gives you a second chance at that. When you dive into a new hobby, you open the door to meeting kindred spirits who share your passion. It's like a cosmic playdate where you connect over something you both love. These friendships become your anchors, grounding you through the tides of change. Who knew that embracing a new interest could lead you to finding your tribe?

Curiosity: The Key to Ageless Wonder

Picture this: you, walking through life with wide-eyed wonder. That's the magic of embracing curiosity during menopause. It's like stepping into a garden of unexplored blooms and breathing in the fragrant air of possibility. Try out photography, take up dance, dive into gardening, or learn a new language—the world is your oyster, waiting to reveal its pearls of wonder. With curiosity as your compass, you navigate menopause like an enchanting adventure.

So let's explore new horizons and let the winds of change guide us towards vibrant passions. Embrace the renewal, let creativity paint your story, nurture your confidence, foster connections, and stay curious like a starry-eyed wanderer. Menopause isn't just about navigating change; it's about flourishing in its embrace. With each fresh interest you explore, you're adding another jewel to your crown of resilience and growth. Cheers to a menopause journey that's as colorful as your spirit!

Chapter 10: Creating a Supportive Menopause Plan

Building a Comprehensive Menopause Management Toolkit: Empowering Your Journey

Navigating the complex landscape of menopause requires a multifaceted approach that addresses the diverse range of physical, emotional, and lifestyle changes that may arise. Building a menopause management toolkit empowers you to take charge of your well-being, proactively manage symptoms, and embrace this transformative phase with resilience and confidence.

1. Education and Knowledge:

The foundation of your menopause management toolkit begins with education. Learn about the physiological changes of menopause, the range of symptoms you may experience, and the potential treatment options available. Empower yourself with accurate information to make informed decisions about your health and well-being.

2. Professional Guidance:

Consulting healthcare professionals is an essential aspect of your toolkit. Establish a trusted relationship with a healthcare provider who specializes in menopause or women's health. Regular check-ups and conversations with your healthcare team can help monitor your health, discuss symptom management strategies, and explore treatment options that align with your goals.

3. Holistic Lifestyle Practices:

Incorporate holistic practices that support your physical and emotional well-being. Prioritize regular exercise, maintain a balanced diet rich in nutrient-dense foods, practice stress-reduction techniques such as mindfulness and meditation, and ensure adequate sleep. These lifestyle practices form the cornerstone of managing menopause symptoms effectively.

4. Nutritional Strategies:

Include nutrient-rich foods in your diet that can help ease menopause symptoms. Focus on incorporating foods high in phytoestrogens (like soy products and flaxseeds), calcium-rich sources, and omega-3 fatty acids. Consider consulting a registered dietitian for personalized dietary guidance tailored to your needs.

5. Herbal Remedies and Supplements:

Explore herbal remedies and supplements that are known for their potential benefits in managing menopause symptoms.

Engage in thoughtful research and consult with your healthcare provider before incorporating any new supplements into your routine.

6. Hormone Therapy Options:

If deemed appropriate by your healthcare provider, explore hormone therapy options. Hormone replacement therapy (HRT) can help ease certain symptoms by supplementing hormone levels. Discuss the benefits, risks, and potential side effects of HRT to make an informed decision.

7. Mind-Body Practices:

Integrate mind-body practices such as yoga, meditation, deep breathing, and mindfulness into your daily routine. These practices can help reduce stress, improve emotional well-being, and promote a sense of balance during menopause.

8. Social Support:

Engage with a support network of friends, family, or online communities. Sharing your experiences, challenges, and successes with others who understand what you're going through can provide comfort, encouragement, and a sense of belonging.

9. Self-Care Rituals:

Create self-care rituals that prioritize your well-being. Whether it's practicing a nightly skincare routine, enjoying a warm bath infused with essential oils, or setting aside time for hobbies you love, self-care rituals contribute to your overall sense of happiness and relaxation.

10. Regular Reflection and Adjustment:

Periodically assess the effectiveness of the tools and strategies in your toolkit. Keep a journal to track your symptoms, progress, and emotional experiences. Adjust and refine your approach as needed to ensure that your toolkit remains relevant and effective throughout your menopausal journey.

Building a comprehensive menopause management toolkit empowers you to embrace this phase with resilience, adaptability, and a sense of empowerment. By assembling a range of strategies that address the diverse aspects of menopause, you create a foundation for navigating the challenges and transformations of this transition while prioritizing your overall well-being.

Tracking Symptoms and Progress:

Empowering Menopause Management

Effectively managing menopause involves understanding how your body responds to the changes it's experiencing. Tracking symptoms and progress empowers you with valuable insights, enabling you to make informed decisions, identify patterns, and tailor your self-care strategies for optimal well-being throughout this transformative journey.

Benefits of Symptom Tracking:

Keeping a detailed record of your menopause symptoms offers several benefits:

1. Identifying Patterns: Symptom tracking allows you to identify patterns, triggers, and potential correlations between different symptoms. This insight can help you pinpoint specific factors that exacerbate or ease certain symptoms.

2. Informed Communication: When consulting with healthcare professionals, having accurate and detailed information about your symptoms can facilitate more productive conversations. You'll be better equipped to describe your experiences, aiding in diagnosis and treatment planning.

3. Personalized Strategies: As you analyze your symptom patterns over time, you can adjust your self-care routine to better address your unique needs. This customization enhances the effectiveness of your approach and improves your overall well-being.Creating a Symptom Tracking System:

To create an effective symptom tracking system:

1. Choose a Method: You can use a physical journal, a digital note-taking app, or even specialized menopause symptom tracking apps to record your experiences.

2. Be Comprehensive: Note the onset, intensity, and duration of each symptom. Include details about your daily routine, dietary choices, exercise, stress levels, and any other factors you suspect may contribute to symptom changes.

3. Consistency: Make symptom tracking a daily habit. Set aside a specific time each day to update your record, ensuring accuracy and completeness.

4. Visual Aids: Consider using charts, graphs, or color-coding to visualize symptom trends over time. These visual aids make it easier to recognize patterns and changes.

Reviewing Progress and Adjusting Strategies:

Regularly reviewing your symptom tracking records allows you to:

1. Identify Trends: Over time, you'll notice trends in symptom frequency, severity, and potential triggers. This information can guide adjustments to your lifestyle, self-care routines, and treatment plans.

2. Celebrate Progress: Recognize the positive changes and improvements you've made. Celebrate even the small victories as you work toward better symptom management and overall well-being.

3. Make Informed Decisions: Armed with a comprehensive overview of your symptom patterns, you can make informed decisions about treatment options, dietary changes, and adjustments to your exercise regimen.

By tracking symptoms and progress, you actively take part in your menopause journey and take control of your health and well-being. This practice fosters a deeper understanding of your body's responses, empowers you to optimize your self-care strategies, and contributes to a smoother transition through menopause, allowing you to embrace this phase with greater confidence and resilience.

Seeking Community and Peer Support: Building Bonds through Menopause

Navigating the challenges and changes of menopause can sometimes feel like a solitary journey. However, seeking community and peer support can provide you with a valuable network of understanding and camaraderie, helping you navigate this transformative phase with a sense of belonging, empathy, and shared experiences.

Shared Understanding and Empathy:

Connecting with others who are also experiencing or have experienced menopause offers a unique opportunity to share stories, insights, and challenges. Being part of a community that understands the physical and emotional trials of menopause can provide a sense of validation and reassurance that you're not alone in your journey.

Validation and Normalization:

Joining a community of peers going through menopause can help normalize your experiences. You'll discover that many of the symptoms, emotions, and concerns you're facing are common and part of the natural menopausal process. This validation can reduce feelings of isolation and uncertainty, fostering a more positive outlook on this phase of life.

Exchange of Strategies and Wisdom:

In a community setting, you can exchange practical strategies, tips, and coping mechanisms that have worked for others. From symptom management to self-care practices, you can benefit from the collective wisdom and experiences of your peers. Learning from others' successes and challenges can provide you with a toolkit of resources to enhance your own menopause journey.

Supportive Relationships:

Building relationships within a menopause-focused community can lead to lasting friendships and connections. These relationships are based on shared experiences and a mutual desire to support and uplift one another. Engaging with a supportive community can help you maintain a positive outlook, enhance your emotional well-being, and provide a safe space to express your thoughts and feelings.

Finding Community:

Seeking community and peer support can take various forms:

1. Online Forums and Social Media Groups: Join online platforms dedicated to menopause discussions. These forums offer a space to ask questions, share experiences, and connect with individuals who understand your journey.

2. Local Support Groups: Look for local menopause support groups in your area. Meeting face-to-face with others who are navigating similar challenges can foster deeper connections and friendships.

3. Workshops and Classes: Take part in workshops, seminars, or classes focused on menopause management. These events often provide opportunities to connect with experts and fellow attendees.

4. Wellness Retreats: Consider attending menopause-focused wellness retreats, where you can immerse yourself in a supportive environment and engage in activities designed to enhance your well-being.

Seeking community and peer support during menopause is a proactive step toward prioritizing your emotional health and well-being. Connecting with others who share similar experiences can offer a sense of validation, empowerment, and camaraderie that enriches your journey through this transformative phase of life.

Conclusion: Embracing Your Menopause Journey

Celebrating Your Strength and Resilience: Embracing the Menopausal Journey

As you reflect on the chapters of your life and the transformative passage of menopause, it's a time to celebrate your remarkable strength and resilience. This phase embodies the culmination of your experiences, wisdom, and the enduring spirit that has carried you through life's challenges. Embracing menopause as an opportunity to honor your own journey is a testament to the remarkable woman you are.

A Journey of Growth and Discovery:

Menopause represents more than just a physical transition; it's a symbolic gateway to a new phase of life filled with potential and growth. Your ability to navigate the changes, both subtle and profound, demonstrates your innate strength and adaptability. Just as you've overcome hurdles in the past, you possess the capacity to gracefully embrace the changes of menopause with resilience and grace.

The Power of Resilience:

Resilience is the cornerstone of your journey through menopause. It's the strength that fuels your determination to rise above challenges, maintain your emotional well-being, and continue pursuing your passions. The resilience you've cultivated throughout your life has prepared you to face menopause with a sense of empowerment, using your experiences as a source of wisdom and self-assurance.

Honoring Your Journey:

As you navigate menopause's peaks and valleys, take time to honor your journey. Celebrate the strength that carried you through every milestone, the resilience that allowed you to weather every storm, and the wisdom that emerged from each experience. Acknowledge your achievements and the unique qualities that define your identity. Embrace the changes with open arms, viewing them as a testament to your strength and the legacy you're creating for yourself and those around you.

Embracing the Next Chapter:

As you celebrate your strength and resilience, remember that menopause is not an endpoint, but a beginning. It's a chapter in your life story that showcases your capacity for growth and transformation. Embrace the lessons you've learned, the challenges you've overcome, and the dreams that still beckon you forward. As you step into this new phase with your head held high, you are a living testament to the remarkable strength and resilience that defines your extraordinary journey.

Reflecting on Your Menopause Transformation: Embracing Change and Growth

As you stand at the threshold of menopause, it's a poignant moment to reflect on the transformative journey that has led you to this point. Menopause represents a profound transformation, not just in your body, but in your identity, perceptions, and understanding of self. Looking back on the path you've traversed and the changes you've embraced, you have the opportunity to gain insight, wisdom, and a deeper appreciation for the evolution you've undergone.

A Journey of Evolution:

Menopause is a reminder of the natural cycle of life, a continuum of growth and change. Reflect on the phases you've passed through — the innocence of youth, the responsibilities of adulthood, and the myriad experiences that have shaped your character. Each experience has contributed to your unique story, molding you into the resilient, multifaceted individual you are today.

Embracing Change with Grace:

Throughout your life, you've shown an ability to adapt, learn, and evolve. Menopause is no different. It's a testament to your capacity to navigate change with grace and resilience. As you reflect on the physical and emotional shifts you've encountered, recognize the strength you've displayed in embracing these changes and integrating them into your sense of self.

A Source of Wisdom:

Your menopause transformation is a wellspring of wisdom. The insights gained from facing challenges, managing symptoms, and nurturing your well-being are invaluable treasures that enrich your journey. Reflect on the lessons you've learned — the importance of self-care, the power of resilience, and the beauty of embracing your authentic self. These insights not only empower you but also offer guidance for others on their paths.

Embracing Your Authentic Self:

Menopause invites you to celebrate your authentic self, unburdened by societal expectations or external judgments. Reflect on the freedom that comes with being true to your own needs, desires, and aspirations. Embrace the qualities that define you, the passions that ignite your soul, and the love you have for yourself. This is a time to unapologetically be who you are and embrace the fullness of your identity.

Reflecting on your menopause transformation is an opportunity to honor your growth, acknowledge your strengths, and recognize the beauty of change. As you look back on the journey you've taken, remember that your story is a testament to your resilience, adaptability, and the extraordinary capacity within you to embrace life's transitions with open arms and an open heart.

Moving Forward with Grace and Confidence: Embracing Your Journey

As you embark on the next chapter of your life, armed with the insights and wisdom gained from your menopausal journey, you step forward with a unique blend of grace and confidence. The transformative path you've walked through menopause has equipped you with the tools to navigate life's changes with resilience, self-assuredness, and an unwavering sense of purpose.

Embracing Your Authenticity:

Moving forward with grace and confidence involves wholeheartedly embracing your authentic self. Menopause has offered you the opportunity to shed societal expectations and embrace your true identity. As you move forward, remember that your authentic self is a source of power and beauty. Celebrate your uniqueness, acknowledge your strengths, and let your genuine self shine brightly in every aspect of your life.

Cultivating Self-Compassion:

Self-compassion nurtures confidence. Treat yourself with the same kindness, understanding, and patience that you offer to others. As you face new challenges and experiences, remember that it's okay to ask for help, to make mistakes, and to prioritize your own well-being. Self-compassion allows you to move forward with a gentle yet determined spirit, knowing that you are deserving of love, care, and respect.

Embracing Life's Adventures:

Moving forward with grace and confidence means being open to life's adventures, embracing both the opportunities and the uncertainties that lie ahead. Just as you've navigated the complexities of menopause, you have the resilience to navigate whatever comes your way. Approach each new experience with curiosity, a willingness to learn, and the knowledge that your journey is a continuous evolution.

Inspiring Others:

This journey is about more than hormonal shifts; it's about growth, evolution, and a newfound appreciation for yourself. Take a moment to recognize the progress you've made, the obstacles you've conquered, and the beauty of embracing menopause as a part of your life story. Your resilience shines through, reminding us all that strength and determination are at the core of your being.

Your resilience, authenticity, and self-assuredness are beacons of light that illuminate the path for those who follow, whether it's friends or daughters. By embodying these qualities, you not only empower yourself but also create a ripple effect of positivity and courage in the lives of those around you.

As you step into the future, remember that your menopausal transformation is a testament to your strength, resilience, and capacity for growth. With grace and confidence, you have the power to shape your narrative, embrace life's challenges, and savor its joys. Embrace your journey with an open heart and a spirit of unwavering confidence, knowing that you can embrace each moment with grace and making your mark on the world.